LABORATORY CADAVER DISSECTION MANUAL

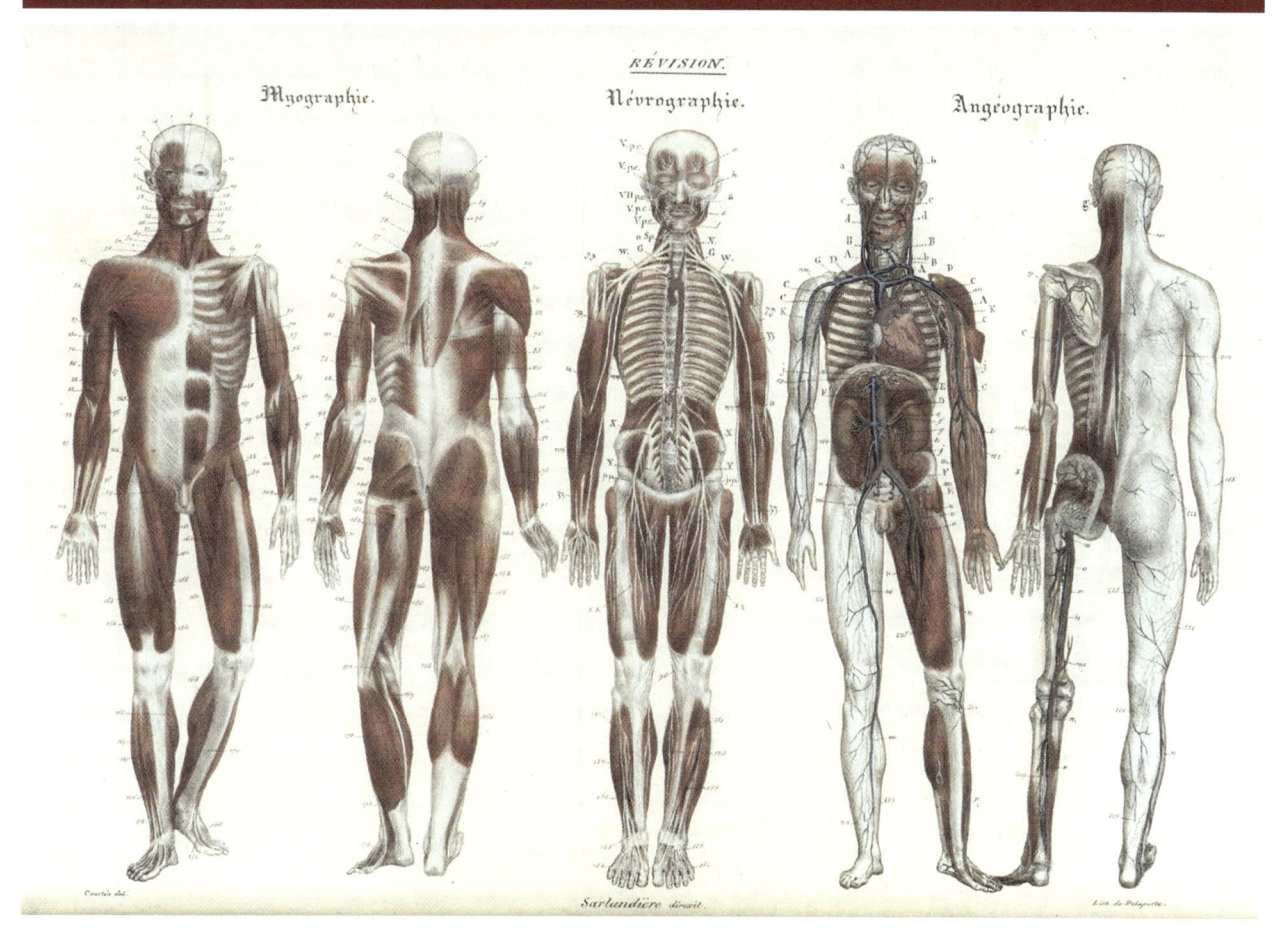

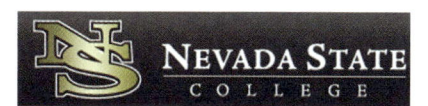

NEVADA STATE COLLEGE

Kebret T. Kebede, M.D. • Hon-Vu Duong, M.D.
Scott Sofferman, D.V.M. • Jill Vuong, D.C. • Vanya Velickovska, Ph.D.

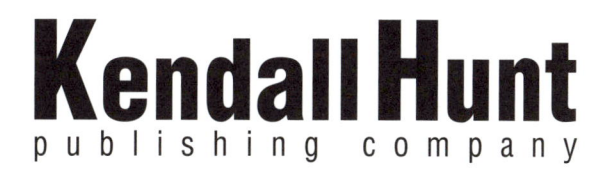

Kendall Hunt publishing company

Cover and chapter opener image:
Systematized anatomy; or, Human organography by Jean Baptiste Sarlandiere and J. Bisbee, 1837.

Kendall Hunt
publishing company

www.kendallhunt.com
Send all inquiries to:
4050 Westmark Drive
Dubuque, IA 52004-1840

Copyright © 2010, 2011 by Kendall Hunt Publishing Company

ISBN 978-0-7575-9178-5

All rights reserved. No part of this publication may be reproduced,
stored in a retrieval system, or transmitted, in any form or by any means,
electronic, mechanical, photocopying, recording, or otherwise,
without the prior written permission of the copyright owner.

Printed in the United States of America
10 9 8 7 6 5 4 3 2 1

DEDICATION

This book is dedicated to the students of Human Anatomy and Physiology at Nevada State College whose collaborative effort and appreciation for learning during the dissection process led to this body of work.

Special gratitude goes to LAS Dean, Erika Beck, Associate Dean Andy Kuniyuki, and Physical Sciences Chair Sandip Thanki for their continued support.

Appreciation and thanks also to all my colleagues who contributed to this work through valuable ideas and collaboration.

> Kebret Kebede, M.D.
> Nevada State College

CONTENTS

PREFACE vii

INTRODUCTION ix

    1. Dissection Using Surface and Regional Anatomy ix

    2. Before You Begin Dissection...ix

    3. Preparing for Dissection x

    4. General Guidelines...xi

    5. Anatomical Terms and Landmarks of Surface Anatomy............................xiii

    6. Anatomical Structures..xiv

    7. Laboratory Review Questions xv

DISSECTION BY REGIONS OF THE BODY 1

    1. Dissection of the Skin..3

        A. Skin of the Anterior Trunk...3

        B. Skin of the Posterior Trunk 4

        C. Subcutaneous Fat..5

        D. Musculocutaneous Nerves 5

    2. Dissection of Muscles..11

        A. Observation of the Ventral Region 11

        B. Dissection of the Thoracic Region...12

        C. Muscles of the Abdominal Region..14

        D. Muscles of the Dorsal Region 16

    3. Upper Extremities 19

        A. Observation of Upper Limb..19

        B. Dissection of the Arm, Part 1..24

        C. Dissection of the Arm, Part 2..25

        D. Dissection of the Forearm, Part 1..28

        E. Dissection of the Forearm, Part 2 29

        F. Dissection of the Hand..34

    4. Lower Extremities...39

        A. Observation of the Lower Limb 39

        B. Dissection of the Thigh 40

        C. Dissection of the Lower Extremities...48

        D. Dissection of the Posterior Thigh..49

        E. Dissection of the Leg..53

  F. Dissection of the Foot 56

5. Head and Neck Region 59

  A. Dissection of the Head and Neck Region 60

6. The Skeletal System and Articulation 63

  A. The Skeletal System: Axial Division 63

    i. Axial Skeleton 68

  B. The Skeletal System: Appendicular Skeleton 75

  C. The Skeletal System: Articulations 83

7. Thoracic Region 105

  A. Observation of the Thoracic Region 105

  B. Muscles of the Thoracic Region 106

  C. The Pectoral Region 107

  D. Dissection of the Mediastinum 109

  E. Esophagus and Posterior Mediastinum 109

  F. The Cardiovascular System 110

  G. Heart Dissection 112

  H. Respiratory System 135

  I. Dissection of the Lungs 138

8. Abdominal Cavity and Digestive Organs 147

  A. Abdominal Cavity 149

  B. The Lymphatic System 165

  C. The Male Reproductive System 173

  D. The Female Reproductive System 175

  E. The Urinary Organs 183

9. Endocrine Organs 195

  A. Observation of the Pituitary Gland (Hypophysis) 196

10. Nervous System Organs and Structures 203

  A. Observations of the General Senses of the Skin 203

  B. The Brain and Cranial Nerves 207

  C. The Nervous System: The Spinal Cord and Spinal Nerves 215

11. The Sensory Organs 221

  A. Observation of Ear Anatomy 221

  B. Eye Dissection 225

RESOURCES AND CREDITS 231

PREFACE

Nevada State College offers a unique opportunity of incorporating cadaver dissection to their Anatomy & Physiology courses. "Nothing beats the real thing" as our students say. It has been an effective tool in laying a solid foundation for their subsequent education in the various health professions. This Cadaver Dissection Manual is published with the intention of guiding students at Nevada State College to prepare before dissection, using their textbooks, models and their classmates before they step in to the cadaver lab as well as to perform or follow dissections of the various regions of the body, step by step.

It is an aggregate of anatomical information extracted from varied sources that we have acknowledged at the end. Since the final editing is done by the publisher, due to time constraints, all suggestions/recommendations in rectifying the errors are welcome. We also intend to have this manual as a comprehensive lab text. We intend to include more challenging questions and assignments to the existing post dissection questions, in the future publications.

My colleagues who have contributed to this body of work are:

Hon-Vu Q. Duong, M.D.

Lecturer of Neurosciences, Anatomy & Physiology, Nevada State College

Clinical Instructor of Ophthalmology, Westfield Eye Center, Las Vegas, Nevada

Scott Sofferman, D.V.M.

Anatomy & Physiology Instructor, Nevada State College

Private practice and Consultant to Nevada Cancer Institute

Jill Vuong, D.C.

Anatomy & Physiology Instructor, Nevada State College

Private Practice-Active Health Chiropractic, Las Vegas

Vanja Velikovska, Ph.D.

Anatomy & Physiology Instructor and Lab Manager, Nevada State College

Kebret Kebede, M.D.

Associate Professor of Biological Sciences, Nevada State College

Consultant level, Specialist List of Orthopaedic Surgery, General Medical Council, London, UK

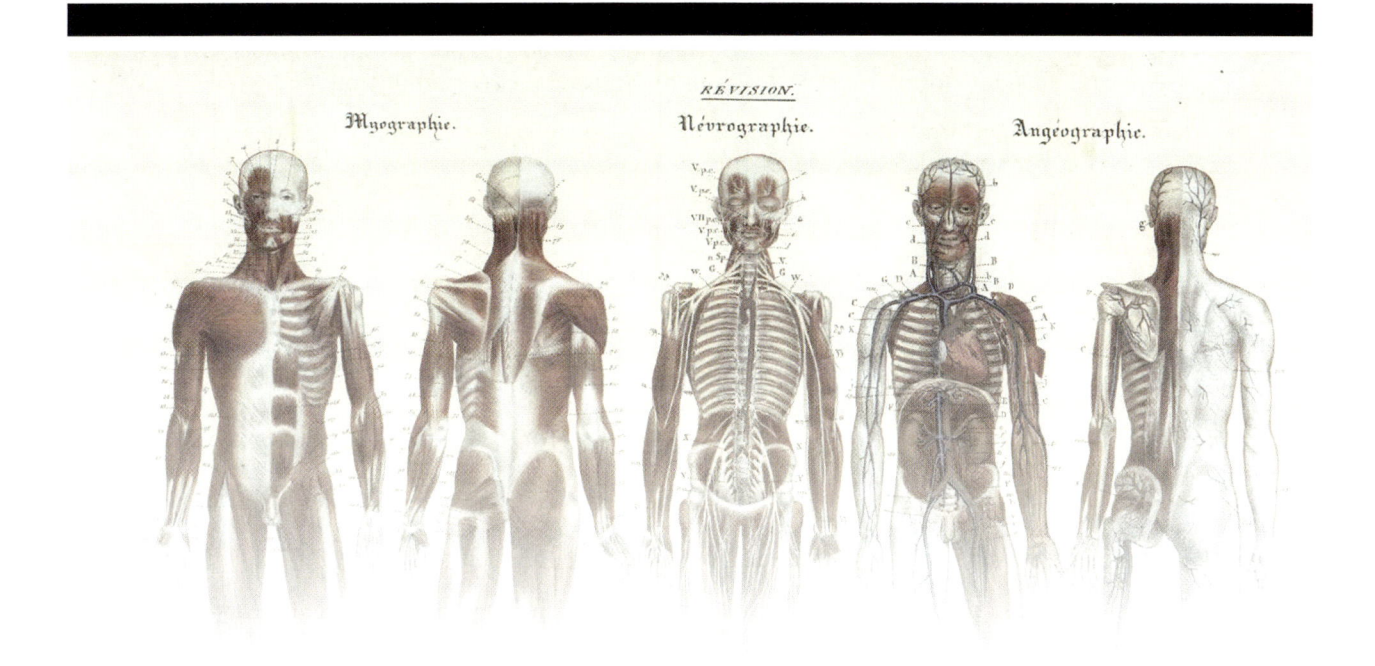

INTRODUCTION

DISSECTION USING SURFACE AND REGIONAL ANATOMY

Cadaver dissection is one of the most intriguing experiences a student of A&P can have. It provides an insight to the structure and, subsequently, the function of the organs in the human body. It is a first-hand experience that exposes what lies under the skin or the outer surface of the human body.

Surface Anatomy deals with the structures, which may be accessed when one dissects a certain area in the body. Surgeons should be proficient in this branch of Anatomy, as should the health care providers who may have to perform various procedures.

Regional Anatomy focuses on the structures that may be found in an area of the body or in a cavity. Observing or studying the organs that are found in the thoracic cavity, such as the heart, the major blood vessels, the thymus gland, and the lungs, constitutes Regional Anatomy of the thoracic cavity.

As we approach the cadaver for dissection, we must observe all the significant anatomical landmarks that are visible on the exterior surface and study what underlies them. During clinical practice the body is referred to in four quadrants composed of imaginary lines going from the tip of the sternum (xyphoid process) to the pubis symphysis and traversing the umbilicus (navel). The second imaginary line traverses the navel (umbilical) in a transverse plane—or from side to side. Dividing the body in these anatomical regions and knowing the appropriate anatomical landmarks allows us to correctly identify the structures under the skin.

BEFORE YOU BEGIN DISSECTION

Remember that the cadavers that are used for dissection come from individuals who committed their body to the study and advancement of science.

1. Therefore we should approach the body with respect and, at all times, ensure the dignity with which we manipulate the body parts. If we are not working on them, the eyes and genitalia may be covered. This is also the case if we intend to dissect in a region for an extended period of time.
2. Students attending/performing dissection should always enter the cadaver lab with the appropriate attire—lab coats or scrubs, covered shoes, hair pulled back (particularly with long hair), and wearing gloves at all times.
3. Whenever dissection is being performed, always remember to hold the scalpel away from your colleagues and maintain a safe area for your movements. Abrupt motion and inattentiveness lead to self- and other injury.
4. If the dissection is of longer duration, masks should be used to reduce the amount of fumes, which may be inspired.
5. Students should wear appropriate clothing for the cadaver lab. Shorts and uncovered sandals expose you to the preservative fluid and body parts that may be dispersed in the environment of the dissection.
6. Students with long hair must have it tied, making sure it does not touch the cadaver containers or the preservative fluid.
7. During the dissection process students have to work together. They may examine the significant landmarks on their partner's body and consult their textbooks to have a clear idea of what they are attempting to achieve.
8. Since students may be using sharp objects, staying focused at all times is mandatory and minimizes the chances for injury to self and to others.

PREPARING FOR DISSECTION

Dissection is one of the exciting experiences in the lab, which is intended to further provide you with a realistic exploration of the anatomic structures.

I would like you to be focused and attentive while performing the actual dissection of tissue because anything you do without appropriate attention can result in unnecessary injuries.

1. Make sure the dissection trays are clean and all the necessary instruments are within your reach.
2. You require a scalpel with a sharp blade and blade remover when you are done with the dissection. Other instruments you will require are:

   Scissors
   Probes
   Forceps
   Ruler
   Dissection pins

3. Do not spread parts of the specimen on the dissection table.
4. Keep all areas in the lab clean with the intent of leaving the space as clean as you found it or better.
5. If you have any injury during the dissection session please inform me immediately.
6. At the beginning of the course you are expected to comply with the lab precaution that was handed out to you.
7. Keep a digital camera and record everything you do in the lab stage by stage. I would like you to forward these images to me via Web Campus. Draw sketches of the structure you are dissecting. It reinforces learning.
8. Use protective gloves and goggles.

*Include a photograph of the dissection kit in the prep room.

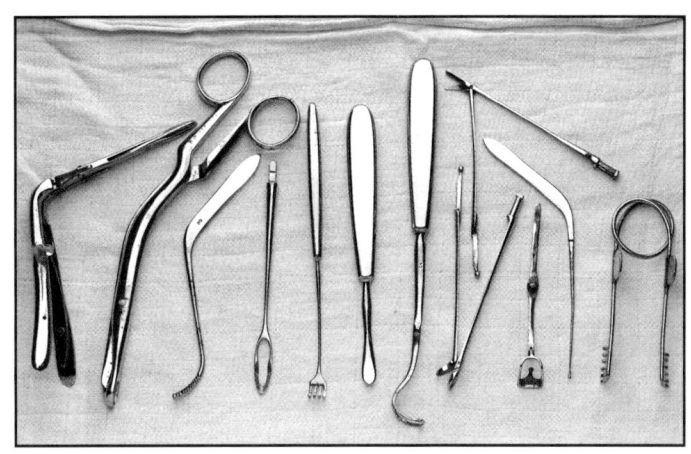

© Milos Luzanin, 2010. Used under license from Shutterstock, Inc.

GENERAL GUIDELINES

Nevada State College follows these general guidelines and requires its students to adhere to them by signing at the end of the statement. Throughout the semester, you will be afforded the opportunity to observe a dissected human cadaver. This process is valuable to your academic experience. However, with this privilege comes important responsibilities. The following are the policies and procedures that will be acknowledged in writing for this privilege. These policies are non-negotiable and anything less will not be tolerated. Any infraction will lead to appropriate disciplinary action.

1. You will treat the cadaver with utmost respect.
2. Cameras, cell phones, or any other electronic or recording devices are not allowed in the cadaver lab.
3. Do not remove any tissue from the cadaver lab. This is not only an ethical issue but, more importantly, a safety issue.
4. Only students formally registered in BI0L 223 and BIOL 224 will be allowed in the cadaver lab. Their instructor will always supervise students, and only four to six will enter at any single time. This means that personal belongings such as cell phones must be secured prior to entry. Students who are not in the cadaver lab must remain in the main teaching lab, which will be locked, and only students registered for that particular class section will be allowed in.
5. While in the cadaver lab, you will wear a lab coat. Scrubs are acceptable. You will wear closed-toe shoes.
6. No one will be permitted in the laboratory without safety glasses or prescription glasses. Safety glasses are available if needed.
7. Eating, drinking, smoking, and smokeless tobacco are not allowed in the laboratory.
8. Formal dissections are to be conducted by instructional experts and, when necessary, specimens will be disposed of in proper containers. Each cadaver tank has its own tissue wastebasket. Waste tissue only from the corresponding tank is to be placed in this wastebasket. Do not put paper towels or other garbage into the tissue wastebaskets.
9. Make sure your waste tissue goes into the basket and not on the floor. Since the tissue is greasy, when it is on the floor it creates a slippery hazard as well as a mess.
10. Following each laboratory session, moisten the exposed tissues of your cadaver with the solution provided in the spray bottles. Then cover the exposed areas with skin flaps and/or blankets. Close the metal container doors. It is to your extreme advantage to do this after each laboratory session. Since we use

your cadavers for laboratory examinations, you will want the best possible examples of structures to identify. Trying to identify dried-out material makes a difficult exercise almost impossible.

11. Place all used scalpel blades in the receptacle located throughout the room. Do not leave blades in the tank or throw them in the tissue wastebaskets.

12. Following these guidelines will ensure a safe, pleasant environment for all of us.

13. Once you have completed your tasks in the cadaver lab, ensure that all of your belongings are accounted for prior to leaving the classroom. Please notify your instructor immediately if your personal belongings are missing. No one is to leave until released by the instructor.

I have read and acknowledge these policies and procedures:

Name _____ Date_____

Tear this page out and give to your instructor.

ANATOMICAL TERMS AND LANDMARKS OF SURFACE ANATOMY

Before You Begin

1. Observe the cadaver on the anterior surface and locate the following: Their alternate anatomical terms are listed alongside.

    1.1 Face and prominent facial bones
    1.2 Forehead (frontal area)
    1.3 Cranium (the head)
    1.4 The orbit
    1.5 The eyes and palpebrae
    1.6 The ear (the auricle)
    1.7 The buccal area (the cheek)
    1.8 Nasal (nose)
    1.9 Oral (oris)
    1.10 Chin (mental)
    1.11 The neck (cervical)
    1.12 The shoulder (acromial)
    1.13 The upper arm (brachial)
    1.14 The forearm (the antecabital)
    1.15 The wrist (carpal)
    1.16 Palm (palmar)
    1.17 Fingers (digital/phalangeal)

2. Moving back to the trunk

    2.1 Chest (thoracic)
    2.2 Breast (mammary)
    2.3 Breastbone (sternal)

3. Further down to the abdominal region

    3.1 The abdomen
    3.2 The navel (umbilical)

4. Pelvis region

    4.1 Pubic
    4.2 Groin (inguinal)

5. Lower extremity

    5.1 The thigh (femur)
    5.2 Anterior knee (patellar)

Introduction   xiii

5.3 Lower leg (crural)
5.4 Tarsal
5.5 Toes (digital/phalangeal)
5.6 Great toe (hallux)
5.7 Foot (Pes/Pedal)

Posterior view of the body

1. Head (cephalic)
2. Neck (cervix)
3. Shoulders (acromial)
4. Shoulder blades (scapular)
5. Loin (lumbar)
6. Elbow (olecranon)
7. Buttocks (gluteal)
8. Calf (Sural)
9. Heel (calcaneal)
10. Foot (plantar)
11. Upper and lower extremities

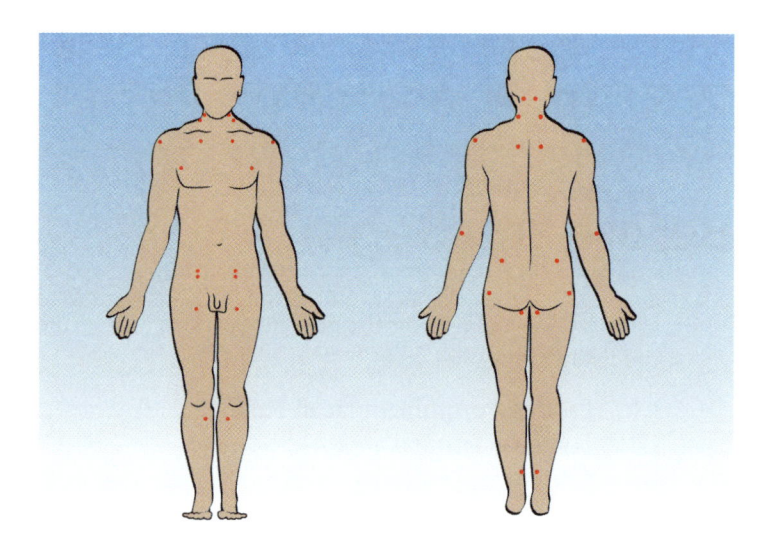

© Kevin Renes, 2010. Used under license from Shutterstock, Inc.

EXAMPLE OF IMAGE OF ANTERIOR AND POSTERIOR PARTS OF THE BODY.

ANATOMICAL STRUCTURES

For all practical purposes, the regions of the body are divided into the following:

1. Head and Neck Region
2. The Ventral Region
    - Thoracic Cavity
    - Abdominal Cavity
    - Pelvic Cavity
3. The Dorsal Cavity/Region
4. Upper Extremities
5. Lower Extremities

Application:

In the clinical setting, if one was to draw arterial blood from the radial artery one is required to palpate the accurate external anatomic landmark to successfully perform the task.

Name: Megan Hartung-Newman

AN INTRODUCTION TO ANATOMY

Laboratory Review Questions

1. Describe the lining of the abdominopelvic cavity.

   A membrane lines the abdomen. It is called the peritoneum, it lines the organs in the abdomen & pelvic region. It provides support & reduces friction within the cavity.

2. What is the anatomical position?

   The body is upright & facing forward. The legs are parrallel to each other. The arms are at the sides of the body, & the palms are facing forwad. The feet are also slightly apart.

3. Define body cavity.

   A fluid filled space in the body that protects & holds the organs in place.

4. If your hand is pronated, what is the position of your palms?

   When your hand is pronated, your palm is facing down & your knuckles are facing up.

5. In what cavity is the heart located? Describe the mediastinum.

   The heart is in the thoracic cavity. The mediastinum houses the heart, thymus, parts of the esophagus, & parts of the trachea.

6. Which structures occupy the dorsal cavity?

   The dorsal cavity houses the brain & spinal cord.

7. Which cavity contains the lungs?

   The lungs are in the thoracic cavity.

8. What is the importance of the Anatomical position?

   The anatomical position provides a perfect reference for individuals talking about the body. It also allows individuals to know exactly what is being described. It is like a universal language.

9. Discuss the difference between the abdominal regions and the abdominal quadrants.

   Abdominal regions are much more specific than abdominal quadrants. The regions include: hypochondriac, lumbar, iliac, epigastric, umbilical, + hypogastric. While the quadrants include the left + right upper quadrants and the left + right lower quadrants.

10. What is a sagittal plane? How is it different from a midsagittal plane?

    A sagittal plane is a vertical plane through the body. A midsagittal plane is a plane that cuts through the midline of the body vertically.

11. List and define the different body cavities.

    There are two general body cavities the dorsal + ventral body cavities. The dorsal cavity consists of the cranial + spinal cavities. The ventral body cavity consists of the thoracic + abdominopelvic cavities.

12. A Frontal place may also be referred to as a ___coronal___ plane.

13. Match the word with the corresponding description:
    a. Buccal
    b. Nasal cavity
    c. Calcaneal
    d. Oral cavity
    e. Cephalic
    f. Synovial cavity
    g. Digital
    h. Orbital cavity
    i. Patellar
    j. Middle ear cavity
    k. Scapular

    _E,B,J_ Associated with the head
    _G_ Associated with the fingers
    _A_ Cheek
    _I_ Knee posterior
    _H_ Hold the eyes
    _D_ Tounge location
    _K_ Shoulder blade area
    _C_ Heel of the foot

14. Locate the term on the image below:

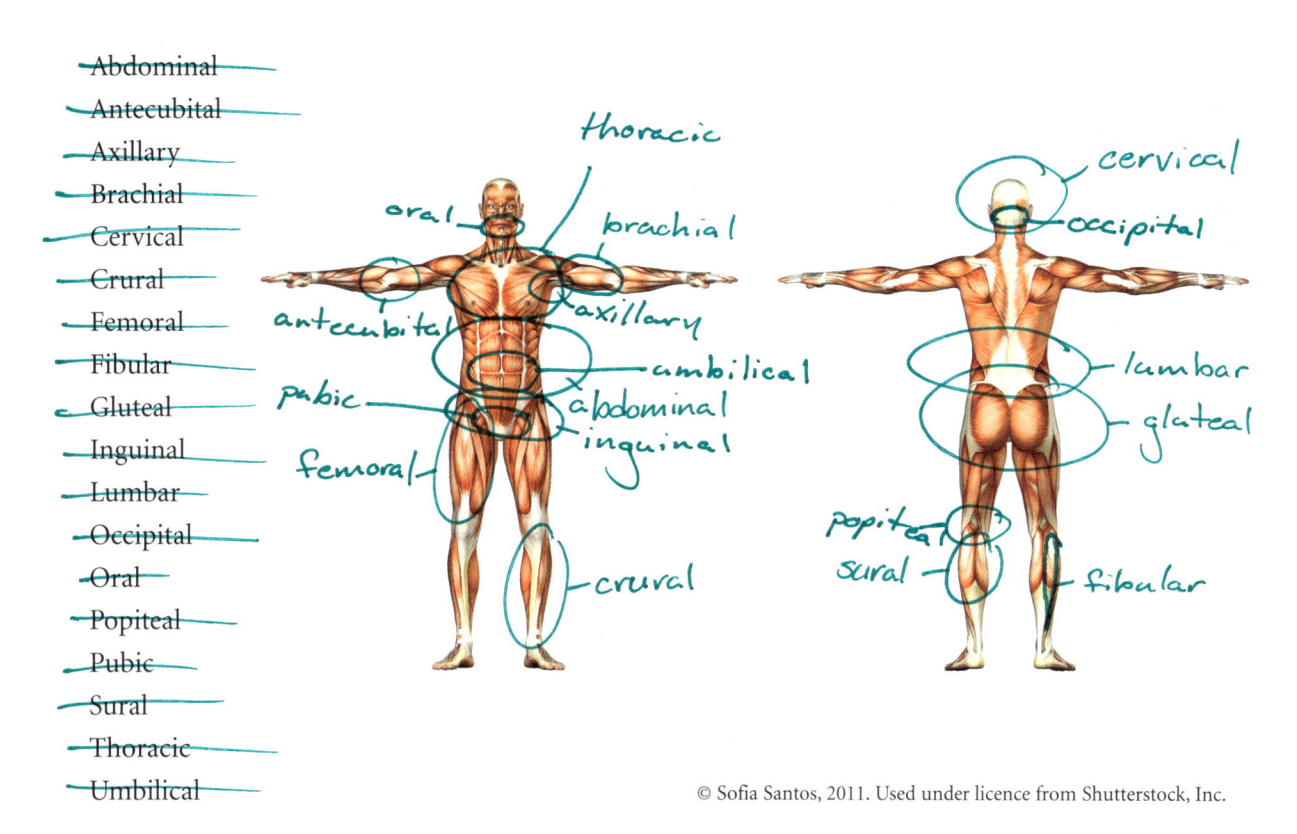

~~Abdominal~~
~~Antecubital~~
~~Axillary~~
~~Brachial~~
~~Cervical~~
~~Crural~~
~~Femoral~~
~~Fibular~~
~~Gluteal~~
~~Inguinal~~
~~Lumbar~~
~~Occipital~~
~~Oral~~
~~Popiteal~~
~~Pubic~~
~~Sural~~
~~Thoracic~~
~~Umbilical~~

© Sofia Santos, 2011. Used under licence from Shutterstock, Inc.

15. Define the Standard Human Anatomical Position

    body standing upright & facing forward, legs parallel to each other. Arms are at the side with palms facing forward.

16. Explain the positional terminology of the following in relation to the standard human anatomical position:

    Face and palms — face: anterior side of head; palms: pronated
    Abdominal cavity — anterior side of body
    Top of the head — superior to the abdominal cavity
    Thorasic cavity — inferior to the head
    The heart — medial to the lungs
    Buttocks — superficial to the pelvic bone
    The elbow — proximal to the humerus
    Shoulder blades — distal to the spine
    Spine — medial to the scapula
    Ears — lateral to the nose
    Nose — medial to the ears
    Heart — medial to the lungs
    Lungs — lateral to the ears
    Fingers — distal to the wrist

17. Locate the nine areas of the abdomen on the image below:

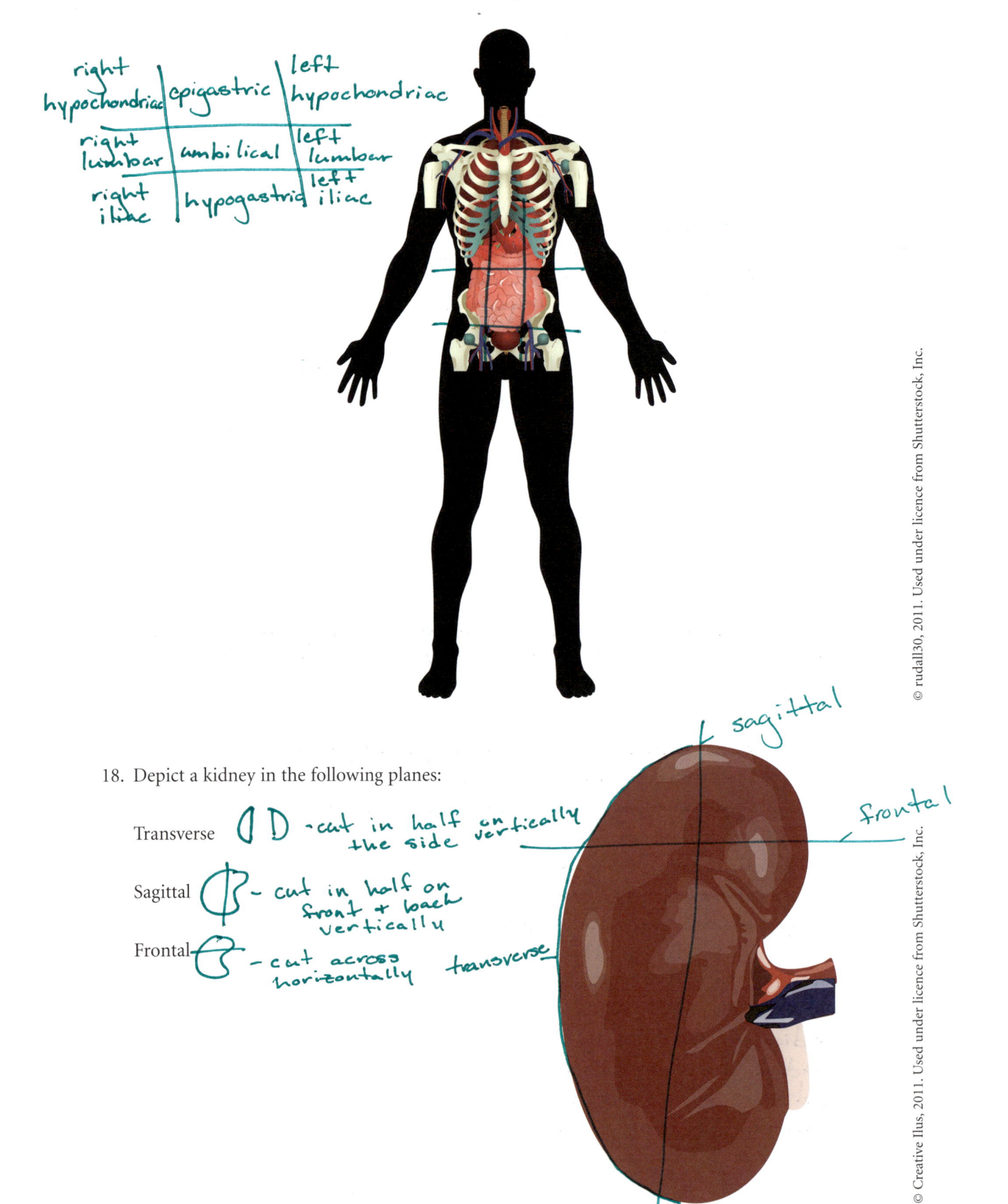

right hypochondriac	epigastric	left hypochondriac
right lumbar	umbilical	left lumbar
right iliac	hypogastric	left iliac

18. Depict a kidney in the following planes:

Transverse ◐ D — cut in half vertically on the side

Sagittal ⊘ — cut in half on front + back vertically

Frontal ⊖ — cut across horizontally

(kidney labeled: sagittal, frontal, transverse)

xviii   Introduction

19. Match the word with the Corresponding description:
    A. Middle ear   C. oral synovial
    B. Nasal   D. orbital

    _C_ Lines a cavity   _C_ encompass' the tounge
    _D_ Secures eyes (anterior facing) _A_ contains anatomy pertaining to hearing
    _B_ Enclosed in the nose

20. Name the following:
    Serous Membrane function _reduce friction by secreting lubricant_
    Abdominal and pelvic cavity bone feature _pubic, ischial, + iliac bones_
    Muscle that subdivides the ventral body cavity _the diaphragm_
    Organ system not in a cavity _the skeletal system_

21. List the cavity name and location for the following:

	Name	Location
Houses the heart	thoracic cavity	mediastinum
Houses the small intestine	abdominal cavity	lower abdominal
Houses the skill and vertebral colum	dorsal cavity	posterior side of body
Houses the ribs	thoracic cavity	chest region
Defined by muscular walls	abdominopelvic	trunk of the body
Defined by belly	abdominopelvic	stomach region
Defined by the multifold protection	cranial cavity	head
Insulating the female reproductive organs	pelvic cavity	pubic region

Identify the following tissue types:

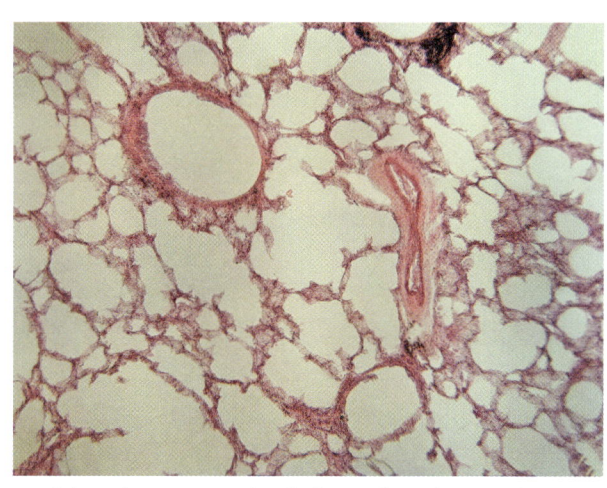

lung

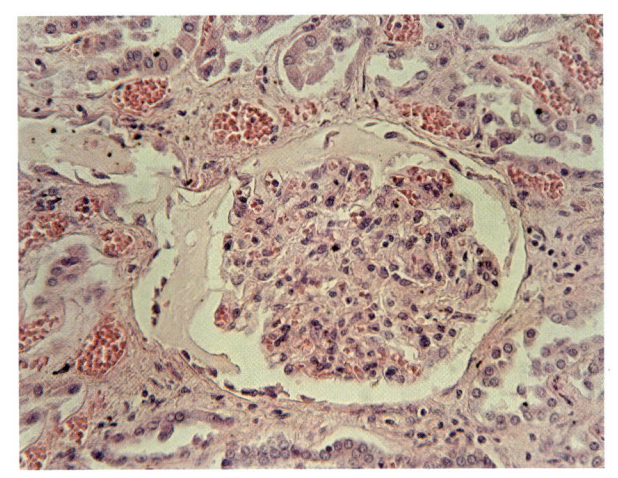

© Jubal Harshaw, 2011. Used under licence from Shutterstock, Inc.

kidney

© Jubal Harshaw, 2011. Used under licence from Shutterstock, Inc.

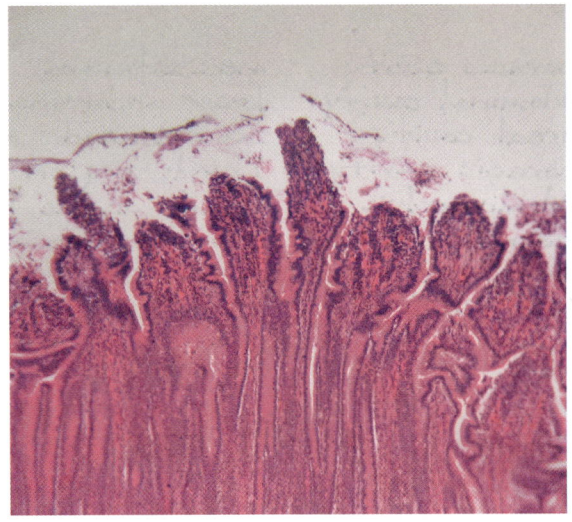

stomach

© Jubal Harshaw, 2011. Used under licence from Shutterstock, Inc.

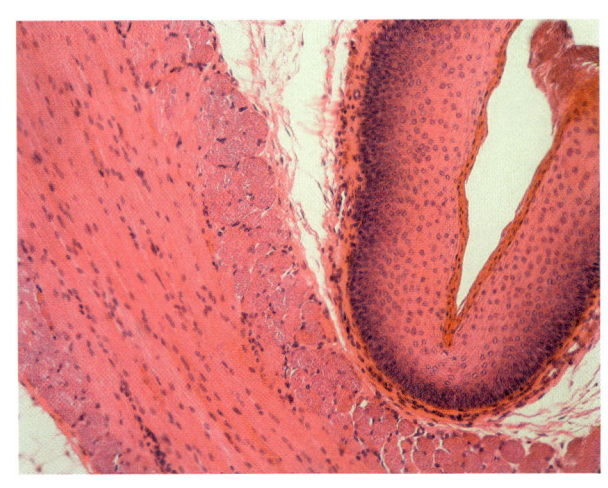

esophagus

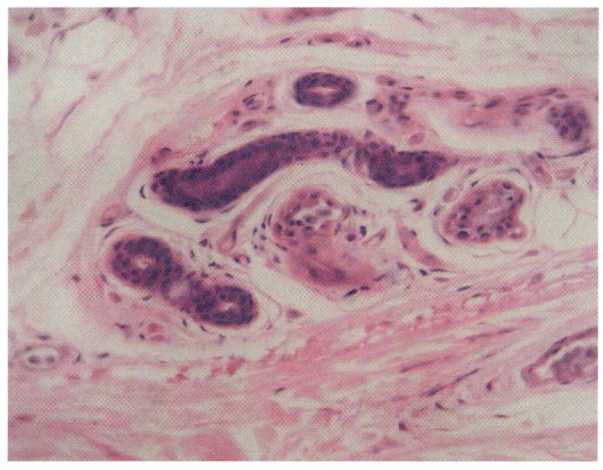

sweat gland

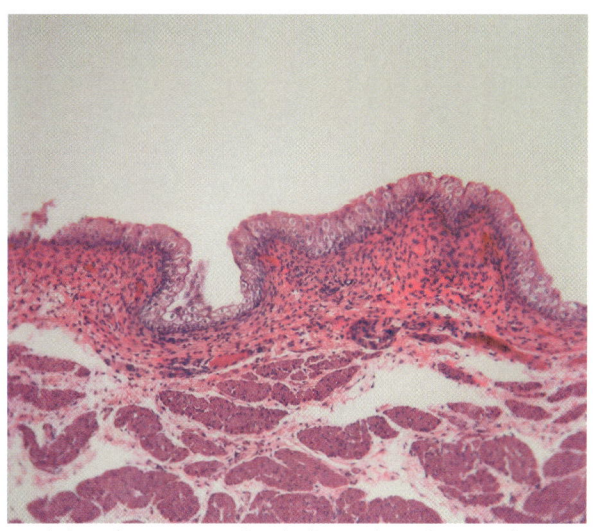

transitional epithelium

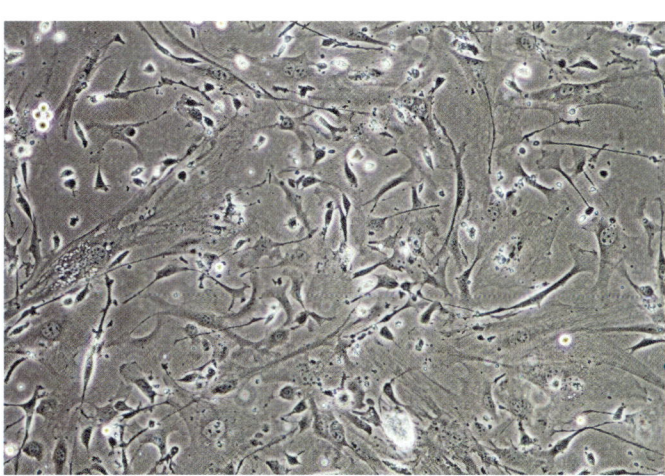

muscle cells, specifically myoblasts

Introduction xxi

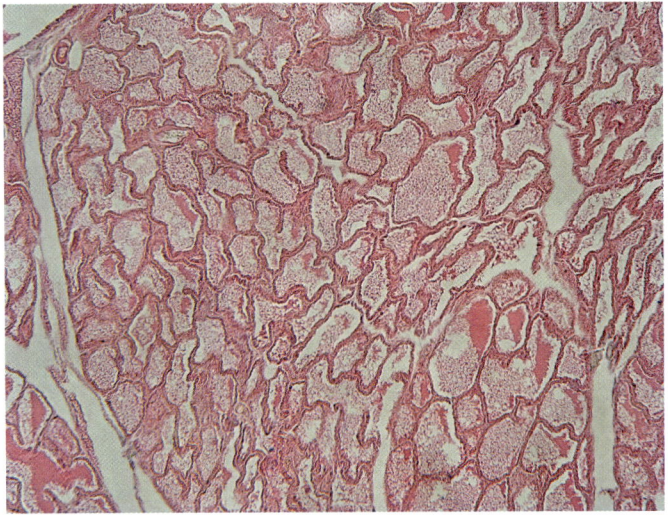

heart

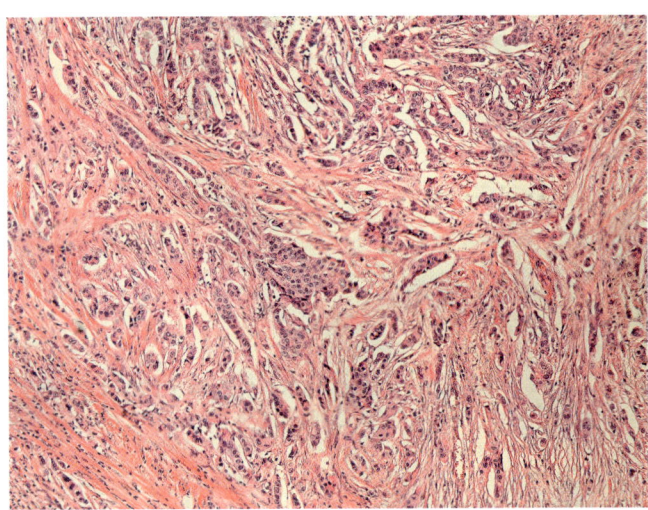

breast tissue

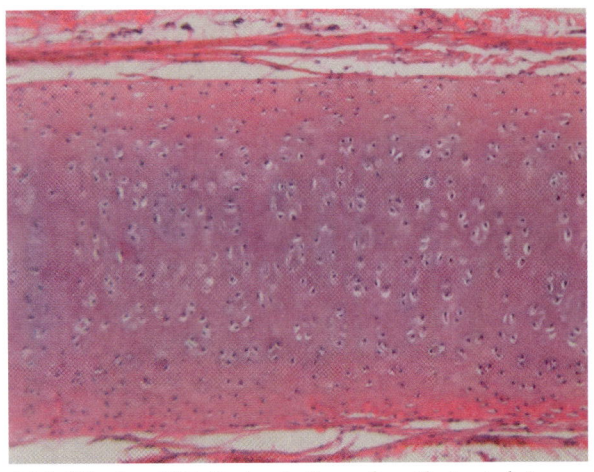

hyaline cartilage

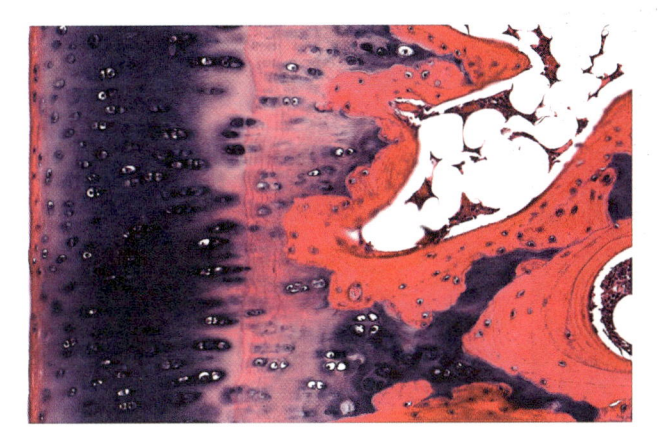

© Jubal Harshaw, 2011. Used under licence from Shutterstock, Inc.

articular cartilage

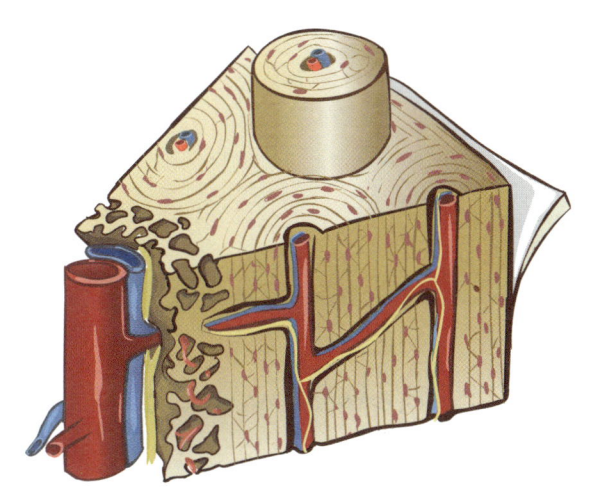

© hKann, 2011. Used under licence from Shutterstock, Inc.

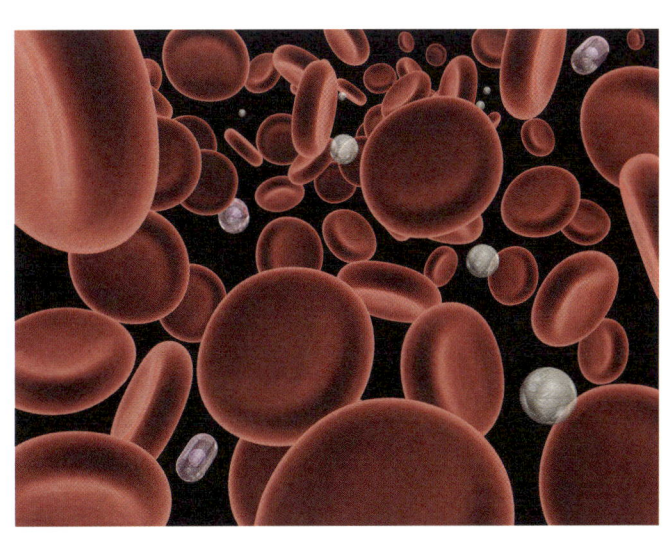

bone

© BioMedical, 2011. Used under licence from Shutterstock, Inc.

red blood cells

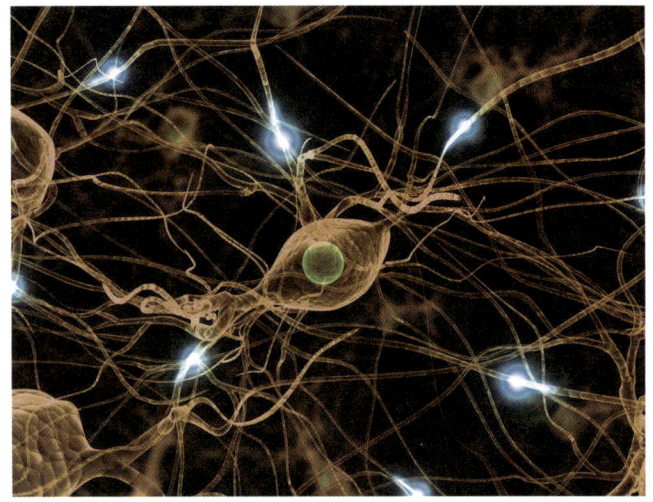

[photo] © Sebastian Kaulitzki, 2011. Used under licence from Shutterstock, Inc. — neurons

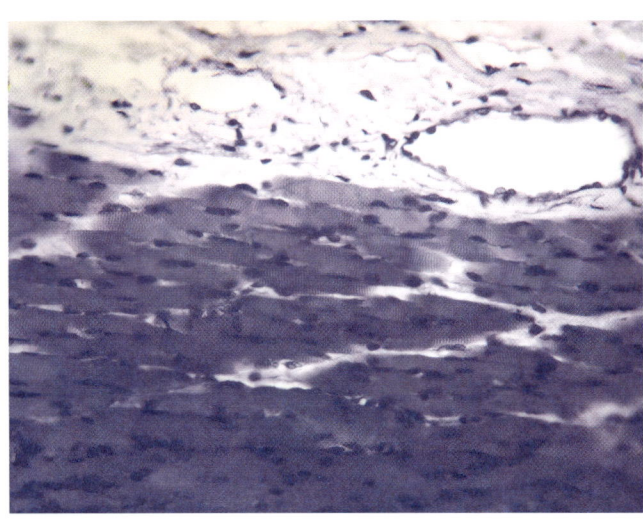

[photo] © Jubal Harshaw, 2011. Used under licence from Shutterstock, Inc. — skeletal muscle

DISSECTION BY REGIONS OF THE BODY

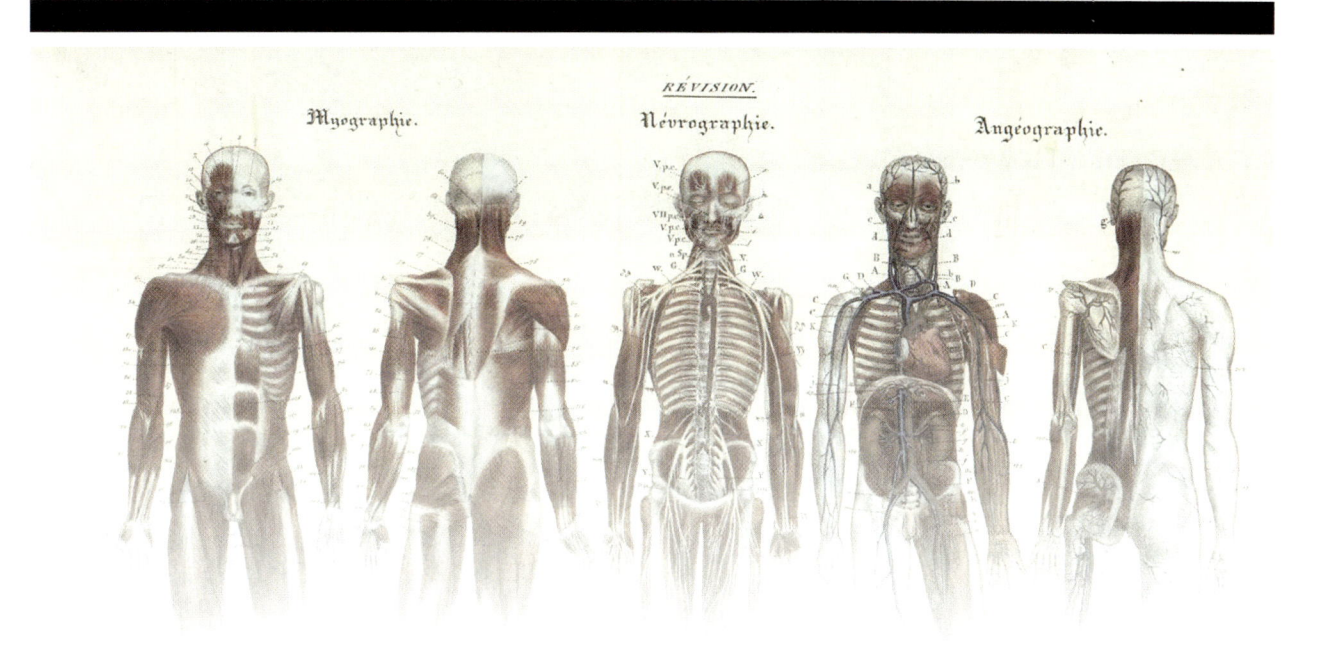

DISSECTION OF THE SKIN

Skin of the Anterior Trunk

Required Instruments
Scalpel Blade size 22 Saw Blade size 10 Retractors Handles 3,4

1. Start by making an incision along the clavicular border meeting at the center of the sternum.
2. Make an incision from the sternal notch to xiphoid process by extending the incision along the body beginning at the manubrium.
   a. Incision must go all the way to the bone, which will cut the skin along with the subcutaneous layer.
3. Continue the incision along the umbilicus to the pubic symphysis.
   a. Gently elevate the skin and the subcutaneous flap to observe that it is anchored to the underlying muscle. These are the cutaneous nerves.
4. Make 2 parallel incisions beginning at the mid infraclavicular area down to the hip.
5. To help students, use several segments to examine skin and subcutaneous layer. The incision can be connected to the transverse incision, which will form quadrants of skin.

Skin of the Posterior Trunk

Required Instruments
Scalpel   Blade size 22   Saw   Blade size 10   Retractors   Handles 3,4

1. Place the cadaver in the prone position with the arms adducted in the lateral position. Palpate (feel with your finger tips) the surface anatomy of underlying structures on the back.

2. Identify the spinous process of the 7th cervical vertebra (C7). Palpate and count the spinous processes of the thoracic vertebrae down to the first lumbar vertebra if possible.

3. Palpate the scapula's borders and the spine of the scapula. In that case, palpate your lab partner's back and identify the spinous process of C7.

4. Palpate the posterior crest of the ilium.

5. Identify the parts of the axial and appendicular skeleton.

6. Study the structure of the thoracic vertebrae using bone specimens that are available in the labs or a complete hanging skeleton.

7. Locate and name the parts of an individual vertebra; using an intact spine on a hanging skeleton. Identify the intervertebral foramina where the spinal nerves exit from the spinal column.

8. **Remove ONLY the skin from the back from the base of the skull to the lumbar region.**

9. Reflect large skin flaps that are dissected from the base of the skull to a level parallel to the iliac crest by lifting the skin with blunt dissection. At this point students should be aware of the presence of cutaneous nerves at various levels.

10. These flaps can be repositioned later to cover the cadaver and maintain the moisture in the back tissues.

11. As the skin is removed note that small vessels and nerves penetrate deeper structures to supply the skin and subcutaneous tissues.

12. Observe intently the small nerves and small vessels to identify the difference in appearance and texture. These small vessels and nerves on the back can be incised during the dissection of the skin.

Subcutaneous Fat

> **Required Instruments**
> Scalpel   Blade size 22   Saw   Blade size 10   Retractors   Handles 3,4

1. As you continue dissection of the skin on the thoracic, abdominal, and pelvic region extend your incision deep down to the superficial fascia surrounding the muscles of this region.

2. The thickness of the adipose tissue varies from region to region.

3. If your cadaver is male or female, the areas that have greater deposition of adipose tissue will differ.

4. If it is a female cadaver, you will observe that there is great deposition on the lateral aspect of the ventral region and also surrounding the mammary tissue. The adipose tissue mass also differs in females of various age groups. The older the cadaver is the less subcutaneous fat you will find. Also note that the adipose tissue is thermogenic and storage for energy.

5. It is different from the visceral fat you may find in the inside of the perotenial cavity.

Musculocutaneous Nerves

> **Required Instruments**
> Scalpel   Blade size 22   Forceps (various size)   Blade size 10   Retractors   Handles 3,4

When you incise down all the way into the subcutaneous layer you will find that there are blood vessels and nerves that are attached to the fascia and throughout the depth of the fatty layer.

When you dissect the ventral region divide the skin into smaller quadrants and each quadrant will contain skin, subcutaneous fat, and the branches of the musculocutaneous nerves. This nerve is important in providing sensory input and can also be a source of pain receptors.

Name: Megan Hartung-Newman   Date: _____

THE SKIN

Laboratory Review Questions

1. What are the accessory structures of the skin?

   Hair, nails, sweat glands, + sabaceous glands are accessory structures of the skin.

2. What is the difference between thick skin and thin skin?

   Thick skin has more collagen + is less elastic. Thin skin has less collagen + is more elastic. Thin skin is usually found in the palms + soles of the feet. Thick skin makes up the epidermis + dermis.

3. What do sensory nerves in the skin monitor?

   They monitor touch, pain, itches, + temperature.

4. What causes the normal color of the epidermis?

   The amount of melanin produced by melanocytes determines the normal color of the epidermis.

5. Why is the skin able to repair itself even after major damage?

   The skin has stem cells in the stratum basale that can form new tissue after a major injury.

6. What are the cells that produce pigment called?

   Melanocytes produce melanin, or pigment.

Dissection of the Skin   7

7. What is the most widely distributed sweat gland on the body?

   Eccrine sweat glands are the most widely distributed sweat gland on the body.

8. Describe the structure of a hair from the starting point of growth within the dermis toward the outside of the skin.

   Hair growth starts at the hair bulb, which consists of the hair matrix. It then extends up through the hair follicle, that is lined with the inner root sheath + the outer root sheath. It then exits the skin.

9. Name the protective functions of the skin

   Physical barrier against mechanical, thermal, + physical injury. Prevents moisture loss, reduces effects of UV, is a sensory organ, regulates temperature, + an immune organ to detect infection.

10. Select all that pertain:
    a. epidermis
    b. dermis
    c. papillary layer
    d. stratum basale
    e. stratum corneum
    f. stratum granulosum
    g. stratum lucidum
    h. struatum spinosum
    i. reticular layer

    __b__ Area that make nails and hair
    __b__ Contains elastic and collagenic fibers
    __d__ Contains melanocytes and merkel cells
    __c__ Contains areolar connective tissue
    __d__ Contains rapid cell division in the epidermal region
    __g,h__ Venue of pre-keratin filaments that are weblike
    __f__ Keratin fibers in a thick skin containing translucent cells
    __e__ Dead cells
    __e__ Dead cells full of keratin that are scale like and shed often
    __b__ Mitotic cells containing intermediate filaments
    __b__ Vascular area
    __c__ Figerprints make in the dermal layer

Dissection of the Skin

11. Locate the term on the below image and notate the role within the skin:

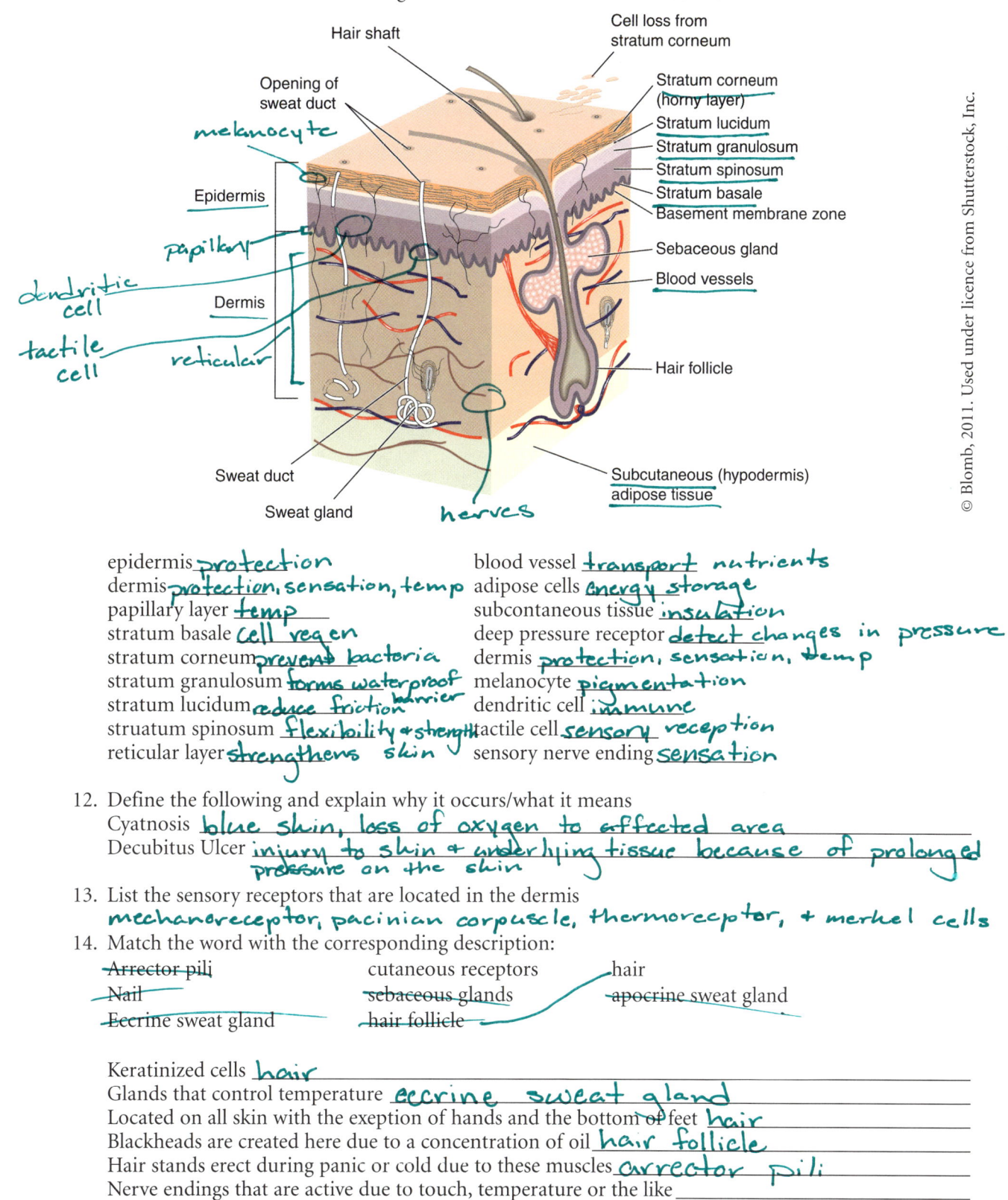

[Diagram of skin cross-section with labels. Printed labels: Hair shaft, Opening of sweat duct, Epidermis, Dermis, Sweat duct, Sweat gland, Cell loss from stratum corneum, Stratum corneum (horny layer), Stratum lucidum, Stratum granulosum, Stratum spinosum, Stratum basale, Basement membrane zone, Sebaceous gland, Blood vessels, Hair follicle, Subcutaneous (hypodermis) adipose tissue. Handwritten additions: melanocyte, papillary, dendritic cell, tactile cell, reticular, nerves.]

epidermis **protection**
dermis **protection, sensation, temp**
papillary layer **temp**
stratum basale **cell regen**
stratum corneum **prevent bacteria**
stratum granulosum **forms waterproof**
stratum lucidum **reduce friction barrier**
struatum spinosum **flexibility + strength**
reticular layer **strengthens skin**

blood vessel **transport nutrients**
adipose cells **energy storage**
subcontaneous tissue **insulation**
deep pressure receptor **detect changes in pressure**
dermis **protection, sensation, temp**
melanocyte **pigmentation**
dendritic cell **immune**
tactile cell **sensory reception**
sensory nerve ending **sensation**

12. Define the following and explain why it occurs/what it means
    Cyatnosis **blue skin, loss of oxygen to effected area**
    Decubitus Ulcer **injury to skin + underlying tissue because of prolonged pressure on the skin**

13. List the sensory receptors that are located in the dermis
    mechanoreceptor, pacinian corpuscle, thermoreceptor, + merkel cells

14. Match the word with the corresponding description:
    ~~Arrector pili~~   cutaneous receptors   hair
    ~~Nail~~   ~~sebaceous glands~~   ~~apocrine sweat gland~~
    ~~Eccrine sweat gland~~ ~~hair follicle~~

Keratinized cells **hair**
Glands that control temperature **eccrine sweat gland**
Located on all skin with the exeption of hands and the bottom of feet **hair**
Blackheads are created here due to a concentration of oil **hair follicle**
Hair stands erect during panic or cold due to these muscles **arrector pili**
Nerve endings that are active due to touch, temperature or the like _____
Contains a cuticle and a lunula **nail**
Covering of the epithelial and connective tissues **cutaneous receptors**
Pubic and auxillary region gland **apocrine sweat gland**
Hair and skin lubricant producer **sebaceous gland**

Dissection of the Skin

15. Locate the term on the below image and notate its role:

Image annotations:
- sloughing stratum corneum cells
- hair shaft
- epidermis
- hair follicle
- dermis
- adipose tissue

- Hair shaft
- ~~Hair follicle~~
- ~~Dermis~~
- ~~Epidermis~~
- ~~Adipose cells~~
- ~~Sloughing stratum corneum cells~~

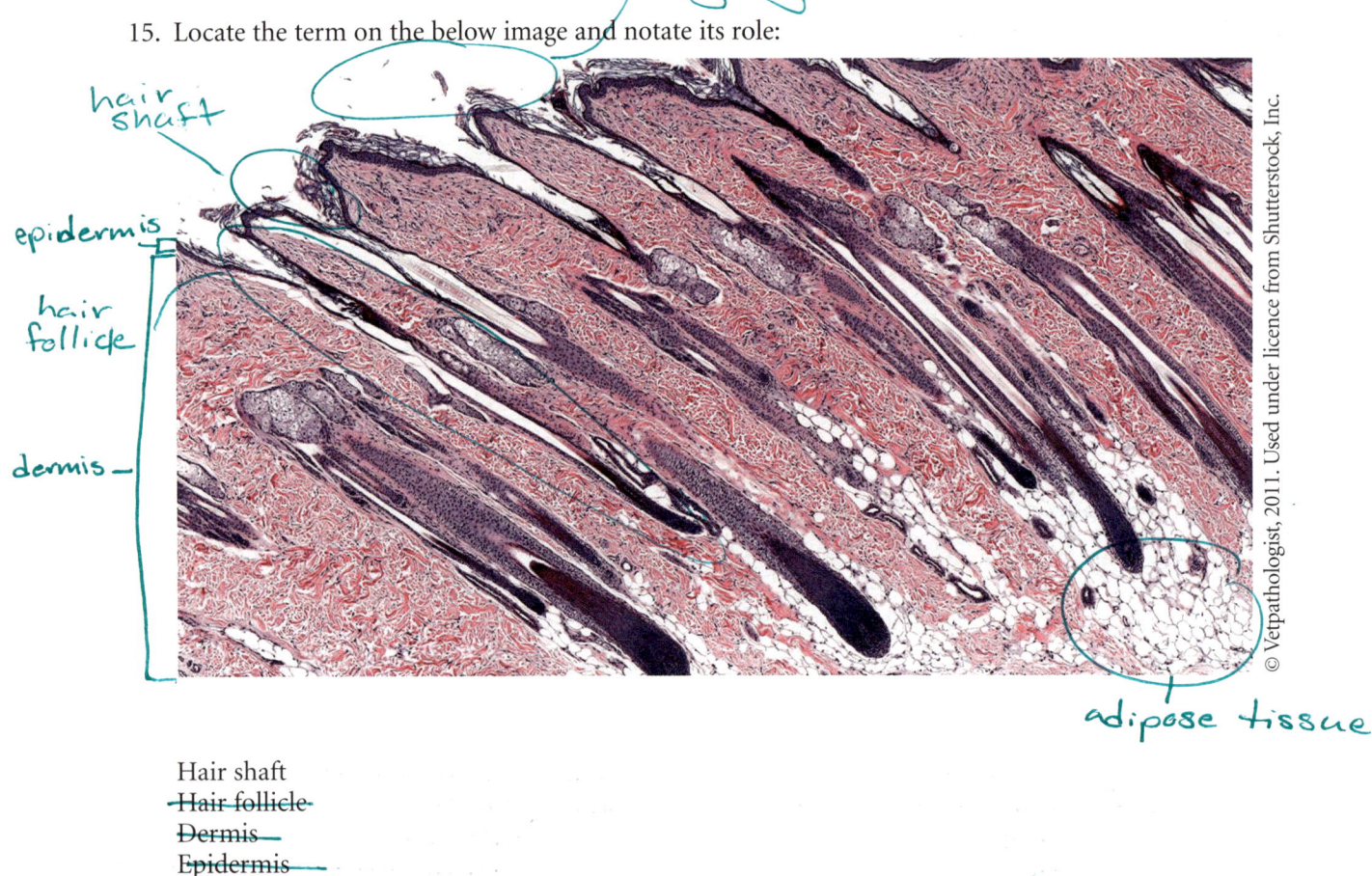

16. List 2 areas of the body that emit a high density of sweat glands, why and what controls its activity

The palms & the soles of the feet because this is where eccrine sweat glands, which are responsible for thermoregulation.

17. List 3 common fingerprint patterns

Loops, whorls, & arches are the three most common fingerprint patterns.

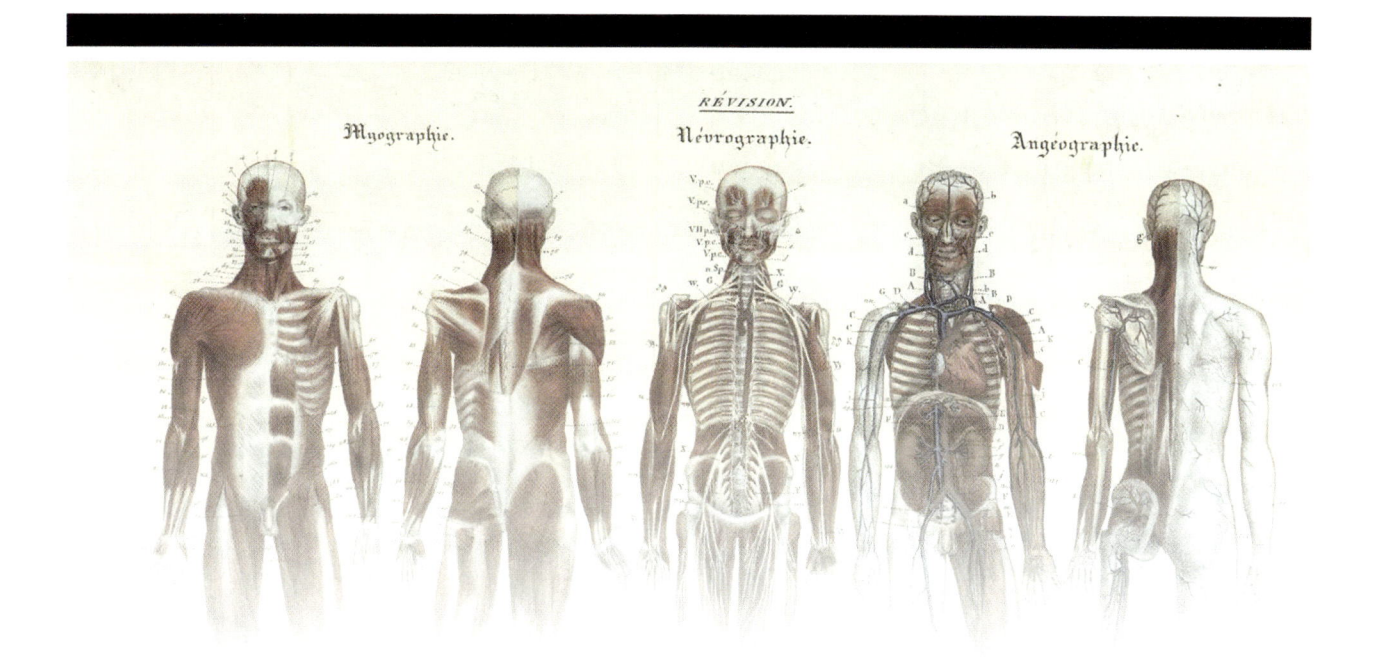

DISSECTION OF MUSCLES
Observation of the Ventral Region
Surface Anatomy and Procedure

PREPARATION

The surface anatomy of the thorax is determined by locating the bony landmarks of the thorax, costal margin, and xiphoid process. Look at an articulated skeleton throughout your observation to assist you in identifying the bony landmarks and points of muscle attachment. The diagrams and illustrations in your book can be a useful guide to help you find the landmarks listed previously.

With your lab partner standing in front of you in the anatomical position, continue to identify the significant anatomical landmarks. Have your partner stand with their arms slightly abducted and extended and estimate the location of each structure. You may use your textbook as a reference if needed. Then locate them on your partner through visual observation and palpation.

Palpate the region of the xiphoid process and notice that it is located in a depression at the inferior edge of the sternum. Palpate the clavicle and notice its curvature. The acromion process can be felt on the superior and lateral area of the shoulder as a projection. You can observe the margins of the pectoralis major muscle on the chest. Have your partner deeply inhale and hold their breath while you locate the costal margin of the ribs. For these excercises it is preferable if the lab partners are of the same gender.

LOCATE

Ventral Region (from Anterior)

- __ Suprasternal notch
- __ Clavicle
- __ Acromion process

- __ Sternum <Manubrium
          <Body
          <Xiphoid process
- __ Sternocleidomastoid muscle (sternal and clavicular heads)

- __ Trapezius
- __ Xiphoid process
- __ Costal margin of ribs
- __ Deltoid muscle
- __ Pectoralis major muscle
- __ Areola and nipple

Dissection of the Thoracic Region

Required Instruments

Scalpel   Blade size 22   Saw   Blade size 10   Retractors   Handles 3,4

1. Start by making an incision along the clavicular border meeting at the center of the sternum.
2. Make an incision from the sternal notch to xiphoid process by extending the incision along the body, beginning at the manubrium.
    a. Incision must go all the way to the bone, which will cut the skin along with the subcutaneous layer.
3. Continue the incision along the umbilicus to the pubic symphysis.
    a. Gently elevate the skin and the subcutaneous flap to observe that it is anchored to the underlying muscle with cord-like extensions. These are the cutaneous nerves.
4. Make 2 parallel incisions beginning at the mid infraclavicular area down to the hip.
5. To help students, use several segments to examine the skin and subcutaneous layer. The incision can be connected to the transverse incision, which will form quadrants of skin.

OBSERVATION OF ABDOMINAL WALL

Surface Anatomy and Procedure

PREPARATION

Before you begin to examine the surface anatomy of the abdominal wall, identify the rib borders, costal margin, xiphoid process, and bone markings of the superior surface of the pelvis. Keep an articulated skeleton nearby during your observations to assist in the identification of bony landmarks and points of muscle attachment as you proceed. Alternatively, you can use the diagrams and illustrations in your book as a guide.

Identify on your laboratory partner, through visual observation and palpation, the surface anatomy of the abdominal wall, using the labeled photographs in Figures 5 and 6 for reference. For you to observe the surface anatomy in this region, your partner must be standing in a pose similar to that shown in the photographs that follow. Estimate the location of the structure, then locate it specifically with visual observation and palpation.

The rectus abdominus muscle resembles a "six pack" on the anterior surface of the abdomen, with the linea alba and the umbilicus as the central divider, and the tendinous inscriptions of the rectus muscle as the horizontal dividers. The external oblique muscles form the sides of the abdominal wall. The anterior superior iliac spines are observed readily when the subject is either relatively thin or in the supine position. The anterior bony part of the pelvis is the pubic symphysis. The inguinal ligament draws an oblique line across from the anterior superior iliac spine to the pubic tubercle. The iliac crest is the widest and highest part of the hips—the part your belt rides above.

LOCATE

Abdominal Wall (from Anterior)

__ Xiphoid process
__ Rectus abdominis muscle
__ Tendinous inscriptions of rectus abdominus muscle
__ Serratus anterior muscle
__ Lattisimus dorsi muscle
__ External oblique muscle
__ Linea alba
__ Umbilicus
__ Anterior superior iliac spine
__ Inguinal ligament
__ Inguinal canal
__ Pubic symphysis

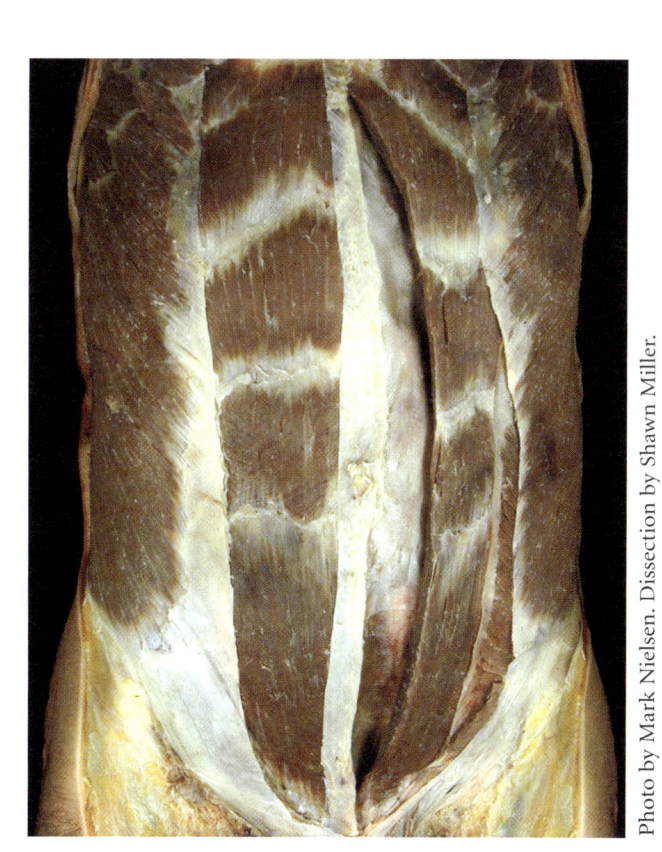

ABDOMEN MODULE

Photo by Mark Nielsen. Dissection by Shawn Miller.

Abdominal Wall (from Lateral)

__ Xiphoid process
__ Costal margin
__ Latissimus dorsi muscle
__ External oblique muscle
__ Rectus abdominis muscle
__ Iliac crest
__ Anterior superior iliac spine

Muscles of the Abdominal Region

Required Instruments
Scalpel   Blade size 22   Saw   Blade size 10   Retractors   Handles 3,4

1. At this level, the skin may have been carefully elevated from the anterior abdominal wall.
2. Continue the dissection by removing all the fatty tissue superimposed on the muscles to expose the fascia surrounding them.
3. The rectus abdominis muscle (the so-called six pack) will be apparent on both sides of the linea alba (White Line), an aponeurosis connecting the two rectus muscles.
4. The umbilicus is at the center of these muscles.
5. Continue by carefully removing the fat and exposing the oblique muscle. The external oblique muscle will appear with its fibers oriented inferiorly toward the inguinal region.
6. The medial fibers will converge toward the fascia of the rectus muscle.
7. When you contine to resect the external oblique after carefully elevating it with a blunt straight instrument, the internal oblique muscle will be exposed.
8. If these steps are carefully completed, you will identify the two nerves between the muscle and fibers of the transverse abdominis; the ilihypogastric and ilioinguinal nerves will be exposed as you observe the orientation of the fibers of the transverse abdominis.
9. By removing the fascia of the rectus abdominis you will also observe the orientation of the fibers that are interrupted by transverse aponeurosis forming the small quadrants of muscle that comprise the so-called six pack.
10. For a wider exposure you may make an incision along the lateral borders of the two oblique muscles and continue the incision superiorly along the hypochondrial margins.
11. Alternatively, you can make a long mid-line incision, which follows the linea alba from the xiphoid process to the pubic symphisis. This deep incision will expose the peritoneum covering the abdominal cavity.

OBSERVATION OF BACK AND SHOULDER

Surface Anatomy and Procedure

PREPARATION

When you examine the surface anatomy of the back and shoulder, review both the bone markings of the scapula and posterior features of the vertebral column. Keeping an articulated skeleton nearby assists you in the identification of bony landmarks and points of muscle attachment as you proceed. Alternatively, you can use the diagrams and illustrations in your book as a guide.

Ask your lab partner to stand in front of you in the anatomical position. Continue to identify on your laboratory partner, through visual observation and palpation, the surface anatomy of the back and shoulder, using the labeled photograph in Figure 4 for reference. For you to observe the surface anatomy in this region, your partner must be standing with arms slightly abducted and extended. Estimate the location of the structure, and then locate it specifically with visual observation and palpation.

On the posterior of the subject, the scapular spine is easily traced medially from the acromion toward the vertebral column, and both the vertebral (medial) and lateral borders of the scapula can be palpated. A furrow over the spinous processes of thoracic vertebrae can be observed to be bordered on either side by the spinalis group of muscles. On the upper back, an infraspinatus muscle may protrude inferior to the scapular spine or can be palpated as a muscle mass inferior to the spine. The rounded eminence capping the shoulder is the deltoid muscle, and its insertion can be observed as a depression if the arm is abducted. The trapezius muscle in the shoulder is more prominent in males.

LOCATE

Back and Shoulder Regions

__ Vertebra prominens (C_7)
        <Superior angle
__Scapula <Inferior angle
        <Vertebral border
        <Lateral border
__ Acromion process
__ Deltoid muscle

__ Trapezius muscle

__ Infraspinatus muscle
__ Furrow over spinous processes
   of thoracic vertebrae
__ Latissimus dorsi muscle

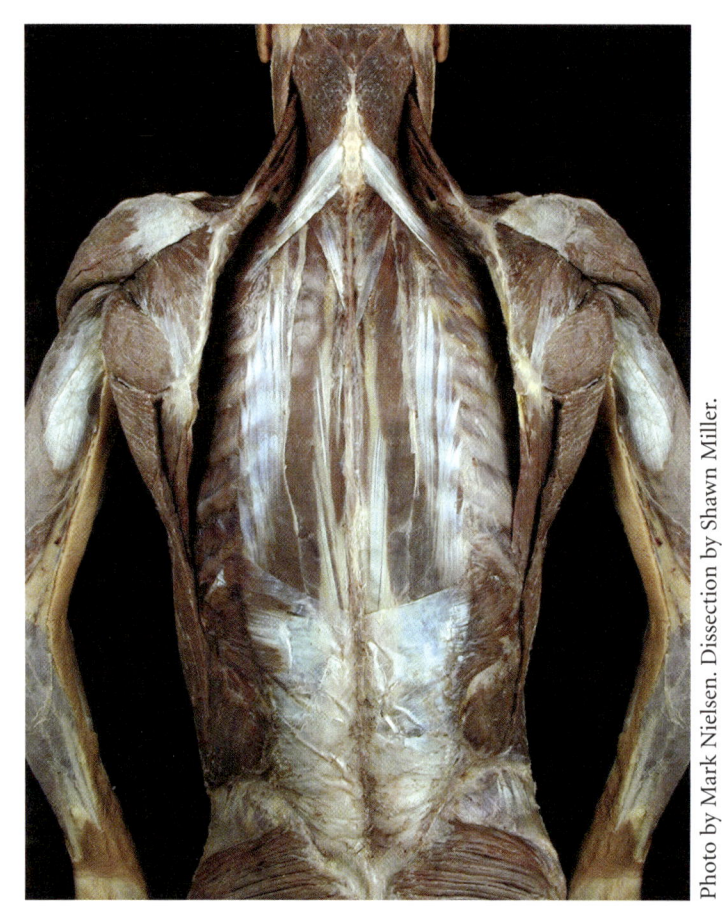

BACK MODULE

Photo by Mark Nielsen. Dissection by Shawn Miller.

Muscles of the Dorsal Region

Required Instruments
Scalpel   Blade size 22   Saw   Blade size 10   Retractors   Handles 3,4

1. For this dissection the cadaver has to be turned in the prone position.
2. In collaboration with your study mate gently turn the cadaver face down.
3. Closely observe the landmarks and the structures underlying them.
4. Start with the cervical region. The 7th cervical vertebra has a significant profusion of the spinous process.
5. You may continue to palpate the spinous processes of the thoracic vertebrae down to the lumbar vertebrae.
6. Notice the prominence of the paraspinous muscle on both margins of the spinous processes.
7. Turn your attention to the scapula. The borders and the spine of the scapula can be palpated.

Dissection of Muscles

Name _____ Date _____

MUSCLES
Laboratory Review Questions

1. The muscles of the pectoral girdle originate on the axial skeleton and insert on the _____ and _____?

2. The biceps brachii inserts on the _____ and the triceps inserts on the _____.

3. What four muscles make up the rotator cuff muscles?

4. What muscles does the Triangle of Auscultation consist of?

5. What muscle is normally used for an intramuscular injection?

6. What is the origin of the pectoralis minor muscle?

Dissection of Muscles

7. Major groups of the appendicular muscles include those of the _____?

8. What is the action of the trapezius muscle?

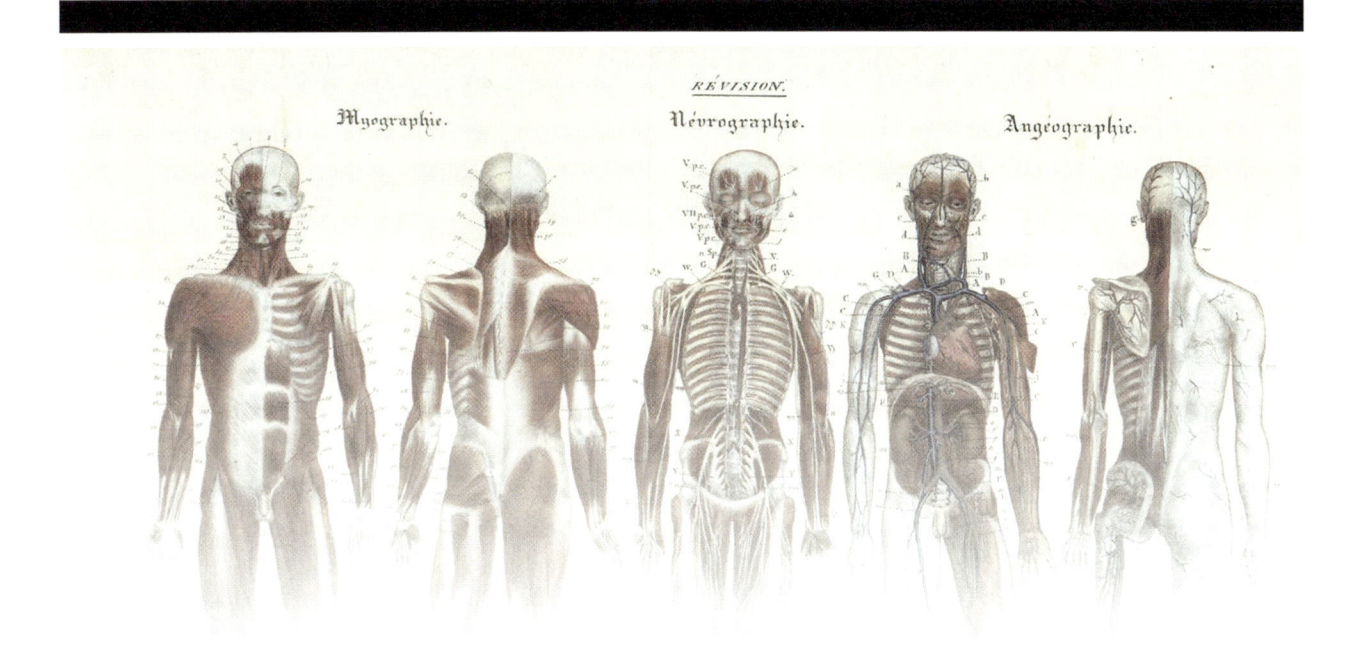

UPPER EXTREMITIES

Observation of Upper Limb Surface Anatomy and Procedure

PREPARATION

Before you begin to examine the surface anatomy of the upper limb, review the bone markings of the scapula, clavicle, arm, and hand. Keep an articulated skeleton nearby during your observations to assist in the identification of bony landmarks and points of muscle attachment as you proceed. Alternatively, you can use the diagrams and illustrations in your book as a guide.

Identify on your laboratory partner, through visual observation and palpation, the surface anatomy of the upper limb, using the labeled photographs in Figures 7 to 9 for reference. For you to observe the surface anatomy in this region, your partner may sit or stand in a pose like that shown in the photographs that follow. Estimate the location of the structure; then locate it specifically with visual observation and palpation.

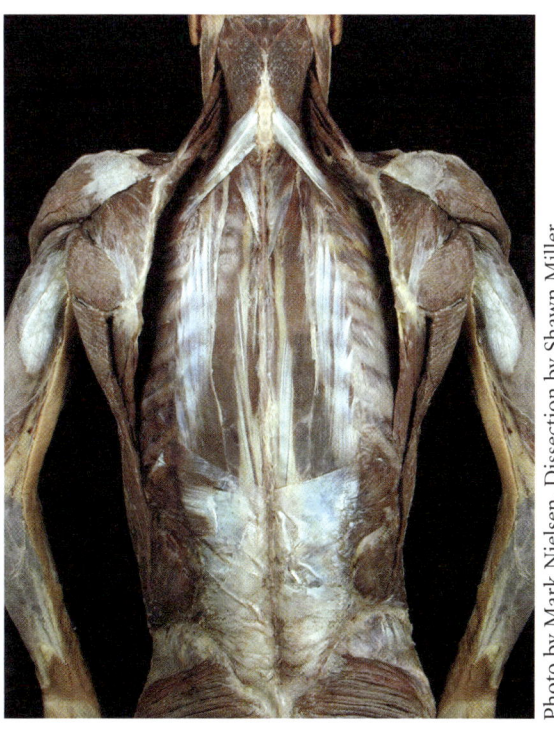

Arm

If you ask your partner to flex their arm the biceps brachii muscle would be clearly visible as the motion is executed. The separate heads of the triceps muscle may be visible with the arm in the extended position and slightly abducted. The cubital fossa is visible at the anterior surface of the elbow between the insertions of the biceps muscle on the radius and the brachialis muscle on the ulna. The median cubital vein crosses the cubital fossa and in the clinical setting is the vein of choice for obtaining blood samples. Just under the skin of the upper arm and over the biceps brachii muscle, the cephalic vein runs superiorly toward the shoulder. The basilica vein runs along the medial side of the arm, just underlying the skin, and disappears near the axilla. In muscular individuals, these veins are readily observed. The medial and lateral epicondyles of the humerus are easily palpated as the greatest width at the elbow. The olecranon process is easily observed. The olecranon fossa can be felt as the "funny bone" when the elbow is flexed. The ulnar nerve lies in the ulnar groove on the posterior of the medial epicondyle, medial to the olecranon fossa, and can be palpated as it crosses this area.

Forearm

The brachioradialis muscle forms a bulge on the lateral side of the forearm along with tendons from most of the superficial forearm muscles (extensors and flexors). These muscles and their tendons are visible at the wrist when the wrist is flexed with tension. Tendons in the posterior side of the hand, when the fingers are fully extended, are those of the extensor digitorum muscle.

Wrist and Hand

The pisiform bone can be palpated at the proximal part of the medial side of the wrist, as can the hamate bone at the heel of the hand, and the styloid processes of the radius and of the ulna on either margin of the wrist joint. The pollicis muscles are visible at the base of the thumb, with the opponens pollicis forming the fleshy base of the thumb, the abductor pollicis brevis forming the flesh pad at the lateral margin of the hand, and the adductor pollicis forming the webbing between the thumb and hand.

LOCATE

Right Upper Limb (from Lateral)

__ Acromial end of clavicle
__ Deltoid muscle
__ Teres major muscle
__ Triceps brachii   <Long
     muscle heads   <Lateral
__ Lateral epicondyle of humerus
__ Olecranon process
__ Biceps brachii muscle
__ Brachialis muscle

__ Tendon of biceps brachii muscle
__ Brachioradialis muscle
__ Extensor carpi radialis longus muscle

__ Extensor carpi radialis brevis muscle

__ Extensor digitorum muscle
__ Styloid process of radius
__ Head of ulna

Right Upper Limb (from Posterior)

<Spine
__ Scapula <Vertebral border
<Inferior angle
__ Infraspinatus muscle
__ Teres major muscle
__ Site of axillary nerve
<Long
__ Triceps brachii <Lateral
<Medial
__ Tendon of insertion
of triceps brachii muscle
__ Brachioradialis muscle

__ Extensor carpi radialis

__ Extensor carpi radialis brevis muscle
__ Extensor digitorum muscle
__ Medial epicondyle of humerus

__ Site of palpation for ulnar nerve
__ Olecranon
__ Extensor carpi ulnaris muscle
__ Flexor carpi ulnaris muscle

Arm, Forearm, and Wrist (from Anterior)

__ Cephalic vein over biceps brachii muscle
__ Median cubital vein
__ Cubital fossa
__ Cephalic vein
__ Median antebrachial vein
__ Tendon of palmaris longus muscle

__ Tendon of flexor carpi radialis muscle
__ Site for palpation of radial pulse
__ Flexor digitorum superficialis
__ Flexor carpi ulnaris muscle
__ Head of ulna
__ Pisiform bone

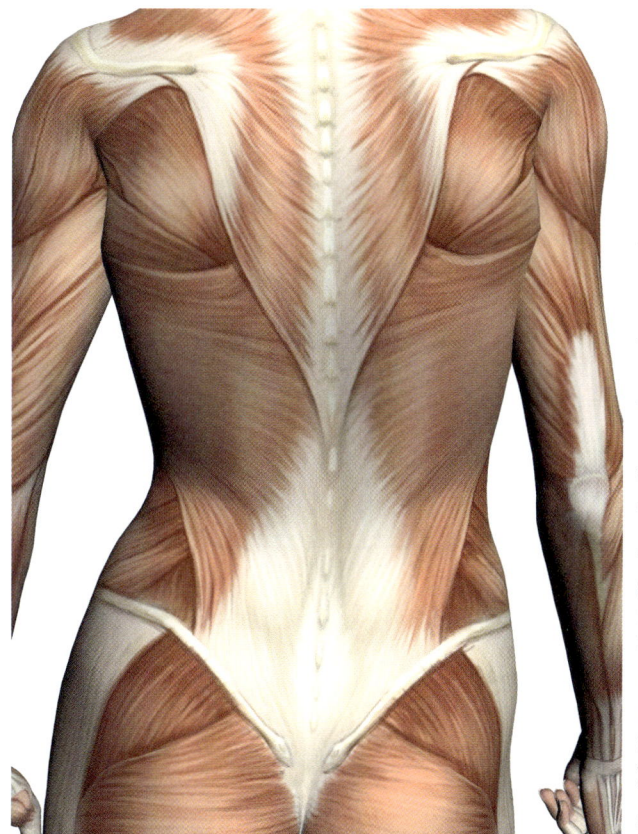

MUSCLES THAT MOVE THE ARM, POSTERIOR VIEW

Upper Extremities

TABLE 2 *Muscles that Move the Arm*

Muscle	Origin	Insertion	Action	Innervation
Coracobrachialis	Coracoid Process	Medial margin of Shaft of humerus	Adducts and flexes arm with the Musculocutaeous nerve	
Deltoid	Clavicle and scapula (acromion and adjacent scapular spine)	Deltoid tuberosity of humerus	Abducts arm	Axillary nerve
Supraspinatus	Supraspinous fossa of Scapula	Greater tubercle of humerus	Abducts arm	Suprascapular nerve
Infraspinatus	Infraspinous fossa of Scapula	Greater tubercle of humerus	Rotates arm laterally	Suprascapular nerve
Subscapularis	Subscapular fossa of Scapula	Lesser tubercle of humerus	Rotates arm medially	Subscapular nerve
Teres major	Inferior angle of scapula	Medial lip of the Intertubercular groove	Extends, adducts, and medially rotates arm	Lower subscapular nerve
Teres minor	Lateral (axillary) border of scapula	Greater tubercle of humerus	Lateral rotation of humerus	Axillary nerve
Triceps brachii (long head)	See Table 3			
Latissimus dorsi	Spinous processes of Lower thoracic vertebrae, Ribs 8-12, the spines of Lumbar vertebrae, and Thelumbodorsal fascia	Floor of the intertubercular groove of the humerus	Extends, adducts, and medially rotates arm	Thoracodorsal nerve
Pectoralis major	Cartilages of ribs 2-6, body of sternum, and inferior, Medial portion of clavicle	Crest of greater tubercle of humerus (lateral lip of intertubercular Groove)	Flexes, adducts, and medially rotates arm	Pectoral nerves

LOCATE

Viewed from the Anterior

__Deltoid

__Pectoralis major
__Coracobrachialis

__Biceps brachii

__Lattisimus dorsi

__Rotator cuff muscle <Supraspinatus
　　　　　　　　　　　<Infraspinatus
　　　　　　　　　　　<Subscapularis
　　　　　　　　　　　<Teres minor

__ Teres major
__ Triceps brachii (long head)

Viewed from the Posterior

__ Deltoid
__ Tendons of rotator cuff muscles

Muscles (Superficial) Viewed on the Posterior Surface

__Triceps brachii, lateral head
__Triceps brachii, long head
__Brachioradialis
__Extensor carpi radialis longus
__Extensor carpi radialis brevis
__Anconeus
__Extensor digitorum
__Extensor carpi ulnaris
__Extensor digiti minimi
__Abductor pollicis longus
__Flexor carpi ulnaris

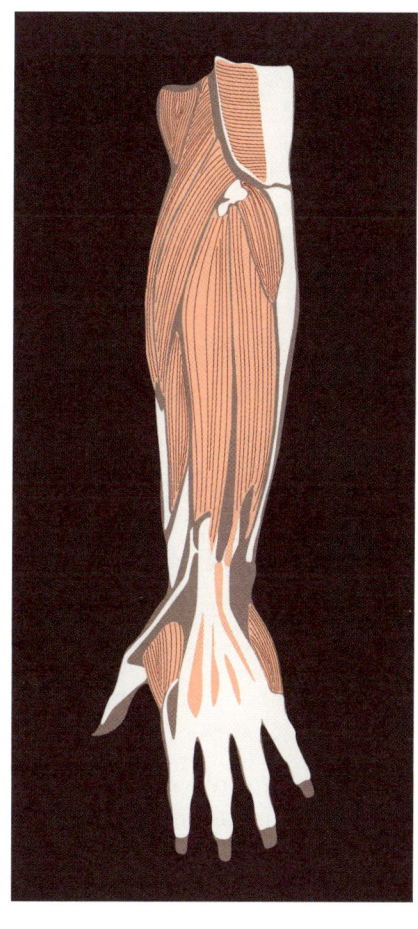

Surface Anatomy and Procedure

PREPARATION

Before you begin to examine the muscles of the upper limb, review the bone markings of the posterior of the skull, cervical and thoracic vertebrae, and clavicle. Keep an articulated skeleton nearby to aid you in identifying sites of muscle attachment as you locate and identify muscles of the upper limb. Alternatively, you can use the diagrams and illustrations in your book as a guide.

Upper Extremities　23

Dissection of the Arm, Part 1

Required Instruments
Scalpel   Blade size 22   Saw   Blade size 10   Retractors   Handles 3,4

1. Incise the skin deeper to the subcutaneous layer and deflect it from the upper arm.
2. To expose the axillary region, remove the overlying skin and subcutaneous fat. This will expose the vessels of the axilla and surrounding lymph nodes.
3. If the cadaver is not a female with a mastectomy, all the lymph nodes should be present.
4. The major vascular branches in the axillary region can be identified. Pay particular attention to the cephalic, median cubital, and basilica veins. The median cubital is the vein usually used for drawing blood.
5. With the arm in abduction, the axillary sheath that encloses the axillary artery can be identified along with the axillary vein.
6. Both the brachial artery and vein are enclosed in a sheath which may be thickened with preservative fluid and will be harder to incise than normal.
7. Separate the two vessels and insert a loop/suture to retract and identify later.
8. The brachialis muscle can be separated using blunt dissection.
9. Identify the two heads of the biceps brachial muscle and their origin. From the supraglenoid tubercle of the scapula where the long head of the biceps originates, continue the blunt dissection to the tendinous insertion in the radius.
10. By continuing to dissect and deflect the skin from the posterior aspect of the arm, the triceps brachii can be exposed. This will expose the lateral head of the triceps branchii muscle and radial nerve.
11. In close proximity to the radial nerve you can also identify the brachial artery.
12. With blunt dissection the ulnar nerve can be isolated at its point of insertion to the posterior compartment as it courses toward the medial condyle.
13. Point out to students the common damage to the radial nerve that accompanies when there is a midshaft fracture of the humerus.

Dissection of the Arm, Part 2

Required Instruments
Scalpel   Blade size 22   Saw   Blade size 10   Retractors   Handles 3,4

1. With the cadaver in supine position and the arm laterally in supination, reflect both the pectoralis major and deltoid muscles.
2. Note: the biceps brachii muscle forms the bulk of the anterior surface of the arm.
3. Explore medially and observe the short head of the biceps, arising from the coracoid process of the scapula.
4. On the lateral side, identify the long head of the biceps, which originates on the supraglenoid tubercle.
5. Note the relationship of the brachial artery and median nerve as they pass along the medial surface of the biceps.
6. The brachialis muscle lies immediately deep to the biceps brachii and can be identified by separating it from the distal end of the biceps brachii, at the biceps tendon.
7. Use blunt dissection with your digits superiorly and note how the superficial fibers of the brachialis connect with the inferior fibers of the deltoid muscle.
8. With the arm in the anatomical position, return to the biceps insertion tendon and locate the brachioradialis muscle on the lateral side.
9. Observe that the radial nerve lies deep between the brachialis and brachioradialis muscles.
10. On the posterior surface of the arm, identify the large triceps brachii muscle, which has three origins.
11. Observe how the long head originates from the infraglenoid tubercle of the scapula.
12. Also observe how the long head extends between the teres minor and teres major muscles.
13. The lateral head originates from the lateral surface of the proximal portion of the humerus and the medial head originates from the posterior margin of the humerus.
14. The long and lateral heads can be separated with blunt dissection using your digits.
15. As you continue this process attention must be paid to avoid damaging the radial nerve and brachial artery, which pass along the lateral head of the triceps brachii.
16. A transverse section best serves in understanding the relation among these muscles, blood vessels, and nerves.

TABLE 3 *Muscles That Move the Forearm and Hand*

Muscle	Origin	Insertion	Action	Innervation
PRIMARY ACTION AT THE ELBOW				
Flexors				
Biceps brachii	Short head from the coracoid process; long head from the supraglenoid tubercle (both on the scapula)	Tuberosity of radius	Flexes and supinates forearm; flexes arm	Musculocutaneous nerve
Brachialis	Anterior, distal surface of humerus	Tuberosity of ulna	Flexes forearm	As above
Brachioradialis	Lateral epicondyle of humerus	Lateral aspect of styloid process of radius	As above	Radial nerve
Extensor				
Anconeus	Posterior surface of lateral epicondyle of humerus	Lateral margin of olecranon on ulna	Extends forearm, moves ulna laterally during pronation	As above
Triceps brachii				
Lateral head	Superior, lateral margin of humerus	Olecranon process of ulna	Extends forearm	As above
Long head	Infraglenoid tubercle of scapula	As above	Extends and adducts arm	As above
Medial head	Posterior surface of humerus inferior to radial groove	As above	Extends forearm	As above
PRONATORS/ SUPINATORS				
Pronator				
Quadratus	Medial surface of distal portion of ulna	Anterolateral surface of distal portion of radius	Pronates forearm	Median nerve
Teres	Medial epicondyle of humerus and coronoid process of ulna	Distal lateral surface of radius	As above	As above
Supinator	Lateral epicondyle of humerus and ulna	Anterolateral surface of radius distal to the Radial tuberosity	Supinates forearm	Radial nerve

LOCATE

Muscles (Superficial) Viewed on the Anterior Surface

__Biceps brachii (long and short heads)
__Brachialis
__Brachioradialis
__Pronator teres
__Flexor carpi radialis
__Palmaris longus
__Flexor digitorum superficialis
__Flexor carpi ulnaris

Surface Anatomy and Procedure

PREPARATION

MUSCLES THAT MOVE THE FOREARM AND HAND

Most of the muscles that move the forearm and hand originate on the humerus. The exceptions to this are the biceps brachii and the long head of the triceps brachii. Both superficial and deep muscles of the forearm perform flexion and extension of the fingers. In the anatomical position, the flexors and the pronators insert and lie on the anterior surface of the forearm, while the extensors and supinators insert and lie on the posterior surface of the forearm. Flexor muscles will be much larger because they are stronger than extensors. The tendons of the flexor and extensor muscles must pass across the wrist to reach the fingers. Two broad, flat bands of connective tissue, the extensor retinaculum, maintain the position of the tendons to the wrist. Just like a bracelet or wrist band, the retinacula aid in keeping the tendons in position as they perform flexion and extension movements of the hand and fingers.

Dissection of the Forearm, Part 1

Required Instruments
Scalpel   Blade size 22   Saw   Blade size 10   Retractors   Handles 3,4

1. Continue dissection of the skin to the forearm using the medial and lateral epicondyles as landmarks.

2. Posteriorly identify/palpate the olecranon.

3. Through movements of the forearm by pronation and supination, observe the relationship of the radius and the ulna. Make an incision along the antibrachial fascia anteriorly starting from the cubital fossa extending distally to the carpal region.

4. By removing the excess tissue surrounding the brachioradialis muscle and deflecting it, expose the radial artery and nerve.

5. Once you identify the radial nerve, observe the superficial branch as it courses toward the carpals.

6. At the radialis fossa, identify and isolate the radial artery and medially the ulnar artery.

7. The deep radial nerve courses to penetrate the supinator muscle and continues to the posterior compartment.

8. Superiorly observe the brachial artery as it bifurcates in to the radial and ulnar arteries.

9. Having removed the skin of the forearm and exposing the muscles of the anterior surface, blunt dissection should now be done beginning at the medial epicondyle to separate the pronator muscle, the flexor carpi radialis, palmaris longus, and the flexor carpi ulnaris muscles and their tendons.

10. On the lateral side, blunt dissect and separate the brachioradialis muscle deeper to the ventral muscles of the forearm to expose the underlying muscles: Flexor digitorum superficialis and profundus, flexor pollicis longus, pronator quadratus, and supinator muscles.

11. Continued dissection of the forearm will allow identification of the median nerve as it crosses the transverse carpal ligament to enter the carpal tunnel.

12. Additionally, you will also be able to identify the ulnar nerve medially of the ulnar nerve.

13. Posteriorly, continue removal of the skin and the subcutaneous layer. As you do this, identify the extensor retinaculum and the synovial sheaths of the tendons entering the hand.

14. At the elbow incise and expose the ulnar collateral ligament, the radial collateral ligament, and the annular ligament enclosing the radial head.

Dissection of the Forearm, Part 2

The upper extremity between the elbow and wrist is referred to as the forearm. The forearm contains flexor and pronator muscles on the anterior surface and extensor and supinator muscles on the dorsal surface. The tendons of most of these muscles (except for the brachioradialis, pronators, and supinators) cross the carpal bones at the wrist and enter the hand.

To Be Observed on Posterior Surface of Forearm:

1. The superficial extensor muscles of the posterior forearm are best observed and identified by working from the lateral to the medial side.
2. Use your fingers as a probe for separating and examining the muscles.
3. With the cadaver in the supine position, rotate the upper extremity to observe the posterior surface of the arm and forearm with the hand pronated.
4. Begin your identification with the brachioradialis muscle, which is prominent at the lateral side with the upper extremity in the anatomical position.
5. Use this muscle as a landmark from which to identify the superficial posterior muscles of the forearm.
6. From the brachioradialis, work in a lateral direction to identify, in order, the extensor carpi radialis longus, extensor carpi radialis brecis, extensor digitorum, extensor, digiti minimi, extensor carpi ulnaris, and the anconeus.
7. Verify the extensor carpi ulnaris by tracing its tendon to the little finger side.
8. The radialis pair is on the thumb side.
9. Trace the course of each muscle and its tendon to the wrist and not the extensor retinaculum.
10. The deep muscle group of the posterior of the forearm may now be examined.
11. Identify the supinator muscle in the area of the cubital fossa by separating the extensor carpi radialis brevis and extensor digitorum muscles.
12. Now identify in order the abductor pollicis longus, extensor pollicis longus, extensor pollicis brevis muscles, and extensor indicis.

To Be Observed on Anterior Surface of Forearm:

1. Now rotate the upper limb to the anatomical position, viewing the anterior surface of the arm and forearm with the hand supinated.
2. The superficial flexor muscles of the anterior forearm are best observed and identified by working from lateral to medial.
3. Begin your identification at your landmark muscle, the brachioradialis, and work medially.
4. Identify in order the pronator teres, flexor carpi radialis, palmaris longus (not present in about 15% of the population), flexor digitorum superficialis, and flexor carpi ulnaris muscles.
5. Trace the course of each muscle and tendon to the wrist and not the flexor retinaculum.
6. Beginning in the area of the retinaculum, each tendon passes through a hollow tubular bursa, as it passes over the wrist and into the hand.
7. The tendon and its bursa sleeve in termed and tendon sheath (or synovial sheath). Observe the four tendons of the flexor digitorum superficialis as they pass deep to the flexor retinaculum into the hand.

Surface Anatomy and Procedure

PREPARATION

MUSCLES THAT MOVE THE HAND AND FINGERS (EXTRINSIC AND INTRINSIC GROUPS)

The muscles of the forearm that provide strength and the basic control of the hand and fingers are termed *extrinsic muscles*. The *intrinsic muscles* provide the fine control of the hand and originate on the carpals and metacarpals. Superficial and deep muscles of the forearm perform flexion and extension of the fingers (as previously described). Again, flexor and pronator muscles are located on the anterior side of the forearm, and extensor and supinator muscles are on the posterior side of the forearm with the tendons of most of these muscles crossing the wrist and entering the hand.

Identify the following ***intrinsic hand muscles***, using an arm/hand torso model or prosected cadaver specimen. The origin, insertion, and action of these muscles are presented in Table 5 and should be reviewed and referred to as you proceed in your observation. View these muscles on the model first before proceeding to the cadaver.

TABLE 4 *Muscles That Move the Hand and Fingers*

Muscle	Origin	Insertion	Action	Innervation
Abductor pollicis longus	Proximal dorsal surfaces of ulna and radius	Lateral margin of 1st metacarpal bone	Abducts thumb	Deep radial nerve
Extensor digitorum	Lateral epicondyle of humerus	Posterior surfaces of the phalanges, finger 2-5	Extends fingers and hand	As Above
Extensor pollicis brevis	Shaft of radius distal to origin of adductor pollicis longus	Base of proximal phalanx of thumb	Extends thumb, abducts hand	As Above
Extensor pollicis longus	Posterior and lateral surfaces of ulna and interosseous	Base of distal phalanx of thumb	Extends thumb, abducts hand	As Above
Extensor indicis	Posterior surface of ulna and interosseus membrane	Posterior surface of phalanges of little (5th) finger, with tendon of extensor digitorum	Extends and adducts little finger	As Above
Extensor digiti Minimi	Via extensor tendon to lateral epicondyle of humerus, and from intermuscular septa	Posterior surface of proximal phalanx of little finger	Extends little finger	As Above
Flexor digitorum superficialis	Medial epicondyle of humerus; adjacent anterior surfaces of ulna and radius	Midlateral surfaces of middle phalanges of fingers 2-5	Flexes fingers, specifically middle phalanx on proximal; flexes hand	Median nerve

TABLE 4 *Muscles That Move the Hand and Fingers continued...*

Muscle	Origin	Insertion	Action	Innervation
Flexor digitorum profundus	Medial and posterior surfaces of ulna, medial surface of coronoid process, and interosseous membrane	Bases of distal phalanges of fingers 2-5	Flexes distal phalanges and to a lesser degree the other phalanges and hand nerve	Palmer interosseous nerve, from median and ulnar nerve
Flexor pollicis longus	Anterior shaft of radius and interosseous membrane	Base of distal phalanx	Flexes thumb	Median nerve
PRIMARY ACTION AT THE HAND **Flexors**				
Flexor carpi radialis	Medial epicondyle of humerus	Bases of 2nd and 3rd metacarpal bones	Flexes and abducts hand	Median nerve
Flexor carpi ulnaris	Medial epicondyle of humerus; adjacent medial surface of olecranon and anteromedial portion of ulna	Pisiform, hamate, and base of 5th metacarpal bone	Flexes and adducts hand	Ulnar nerve
Palmaris longus	Medial epicondyle of humerus	Palmar aponeurosis and flexor retinaculum	Flexes hand	Median nerve
Extensors				
Extensor carpi Radialis, longus brevis	Lateral supracondylar ridge of humerus Lateral epicondyle of humerus	Base of 2nd metacarpal Base of 3rd metacarpal	Extends and abducts hand As above	Radial nerve As above
Extensor carpi ulnaris	Lateral epicondyle of humerus; adjacent dorsal Surface to ulna	Base of 5th metacarpal	Extends and adducts hand	Deep radial nerve

Muscles (Deep) Viewed on the Anterior Surface
__Flexor digitorum profundus
__Flexor pollicis longus
__Pronator quadratus

Muscles (Deep) Viewed on the Posterior Surface
__Anconeus
__Supinator
__Abductor pollicis longus
__Extensor pollicis longus
__Extensor pollicis brevis
__Extensor indicis
__Tendons of extensor digitorum
__Tendons of extensor digiti minimi

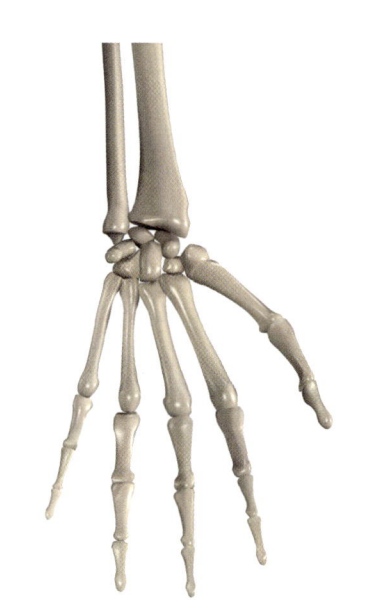

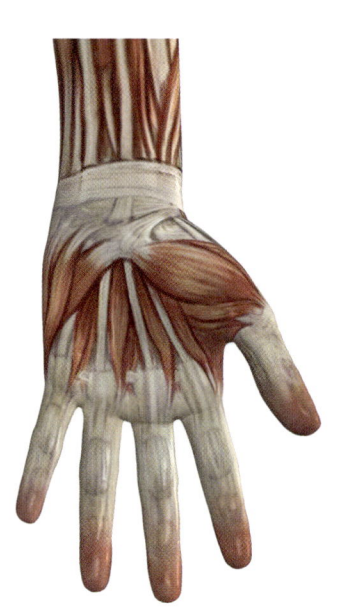

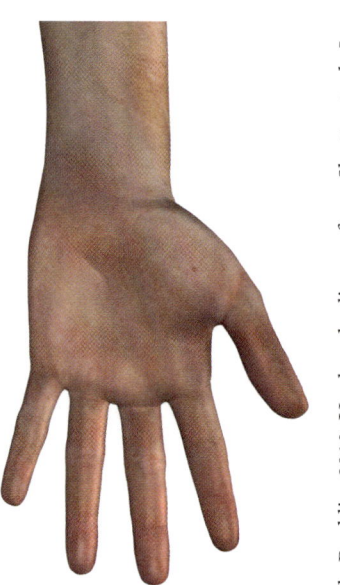

MUSCLES THAT MOVE THE HAND AND FINGERS

TABLE 5 *Intrinsic Muscles of the Hand*

Muscle	Origin	Insertion	Action	Innervation
Adductor pollicis	Metacarpal and carpal bones	Proximal phalanx of thumb	Adducts thumb	Ulnar nerve, deep branch
Opponens pollicis Palmaris brevis	Trapezium Palmar aponeurosis	First metacarpal bone Skin of medial border of hand	Opposition of thumb moves skin on medial border toward midline of palm	Median nerve Ulnar nerve, superficial branch
Abductor digiti minimi	Pisiform bone	Proximal phalanx of little finger	Abducts little finger and flexes its Proximal phalanx	Ulnar nerve, deep branch
Abductor pollicus brevis	Transverse carpal ligament, scaphoid bone and trapezium	Radial side of the base of the proximal phalanx of the thumb	Abducts the thumb	Median nerve
Flexor pollicis brevis*	Flexor retinaculum trapezium, capltate bone and ulnar side of first metacarpal bone	Ulnar side of the proximal phalanx of the thumb	Flexes and adducts the thumb	Branches of median and ulnar nerves
Flexor digiti minimi brevis	Hamate bone	Proximal phalanx of little finger	Flexes little finger	Ulnar nerve, deep branch
Opponens digiti minimi	Hamate bone	Fifth metacarpal	Opposition of fifth metacarpal bone	Ulnar nerve, deep branch
Lumbricals (4)	Tendons of flexor digitorum profundus	Tendons of extensor digitomm	Flexes metacarpophalangeal joints, extends middle and distal phalanges	#1 and #2 by median nerve, #3 and #4 by ulnar nerve, deep branch
Dorsal Interossei	Each originates from opposing faces of two metacarpal bones (I and II, II and III, III and IV, IV and V)	Bases of proximal phalanges of fngers 2-4	Abduct fingers 2-4 away from the midline axis of the middle finger (3), flex Metacarpophalangeal Joints, extends fingertips	Ulnar nerve deep branch
Palmar Interossei	Sides of metacarpal bones II, IV, and V	Bases of proximal phalanges of fingers 2, 4 and 5	Adduct fingers 2, 4 and 5 toward the midline axis of the middle finger (3), flex metacarpophalangeal joints, extend fingertips	Ulnar nerve deep branch

Upper Extremities

Intrinsic Muscles of the Hand (Anterior and Posterior Views)

__Abductor pollicis brevis
__Adductor pollicis
__Opponens pollicis
__Palmaris brevis
__Abductor digiti minimi
__Flexor digiti minimi brevis
__Opponens digiti minimi
__Lumbricals (4)
__Dorsal interossei (4)
__Palmar inerossei (3)
__Flexor pollicis brevis

LOCATE

Extrinsic Muscles of the Hand (Anterior and Posterior Views)

__Flexor digitorum superficialis
__Flexor digitorum profundus
__Flexor pollicis longus
__Abductor pollicis longus
__Extensor digitorum
__Extensor retinaculum
__Flexor retinaculum
__Extensor pollicis brevis
__Extensor pollicis longus

Dissection of the Hand

Required Instruments
Scalpel   Blade size 22   Saw   Blade size 10   Retractors   Handles 3,4

1. On skeletal material identify the carpal bones and their anatomical positioning. Observe their articulations with the radius and ulna as well as with the metacarpal bones.

2. Identify the carpal, metacarpal, metacarpal-phalangeal, proximal, and distal interphalangeal joints. Specifically identify the extent and attachments of the flexor retinaculum on the ventral surface of the hand. This participates in forming the carpal tunnel, through which passes the tendons of the flexor digitorum superficialis and flexor digitorum profundus and flexor pollicis longus muscles as well as the median nerve.

3. Start hand dissection on the dorsal surface after removal of the skin. Dissect the long extensor tendons to each digit and free them from their extensor expansions en route to the distal aspects of each finger.

4. Move them aside and dissect and identify the four dorsal interossei muscles between the metacarpals by cleaning their margins. Follow the radial and ulnar contributions to the dorsal carpal arch. All non-muscular structures on this dorsal surface lie very superficially.

5. Clean the radial artery and follow it into the region of the first dorsal interosseous muscle after giving off its superficial branch. Remove the skin and fascia of the hand. Make longitudinal incisions to the ends of each digit through the fibrous digital sheath using a scissors to release the tendons of the flexor digitorum superficialis and flexor digitorum profundus muscles. **Do not cut the tendons in the hand.**

6. Cut the flexor retinaculum proximally distally exposing the contents of the carpal tunnel.

7. Dissect the median nerve in this compartment and identify the recurrent median branch of the median nerve entering the thenar eminence distal to the flexor retinaculum.

8. Follow the ulnar artery into the palm and clean the deep branch of the ulnar artery lying at the lateral aspect of the flexor retinaculum. Proximal to the flexor retinaculum locate and dissect the superficial branch of the radial artery and the continuation of the radial artery as it dives deep to the thenar muscles (and continues into formation of the deep palmer arch).

9. Dissect the superficial palmer arch and its branches (common palmer digital), branches of the ulnar nerve, and additional branches of the median nerve.

10. Dissect the fascia overlying the thenar muscle group and identify the thenar muscles: flexor pollicis brevis, abductor pollicis brevis, and opponens pollicis. Clean the margins and tendinous components of each muscle.

11. Deep and distal to the thenar muscles dissect the two heads of the adductor pollicis muscle, transverse and oblique.

12. Dissect the fascia overlying the hypothenar muscle group and identify the hypothenar muscles: flexor digiti minimi, abductor digiti minimi, and opponens digiti minimi. Clean the margins and tendinous components of each muscle.

13. Deep to the branches of the median nerve dissect the deep palmer arterial arch lying across the metacarpals distal to their bases. Clean the palmer metacarpal arteries that run distally and anastomose with the common palmer digital arteries from the superficial palmer arch.

14. Dissect the princeps pollicis and radialis indicis arteries arising between the first and second metacarpals.

15. Identify the four lumbrical muscles arising from the tendons of the flexor digitorum profundus. Deep to these lie the three palmer interosseous muscles originating on metacarpals and inserting on proximal phalanges.

Name _____ Date _____

UPPER EXTREMITIES
Laboratory Review Questions

1. The muscles that cause pronation of the forearm include?

2. What are the muscles of the upper arm?

3. The muscle that can adduct, flex, and extend the arm is the _____?

4. Which cell type is responsible for skeletal muscle regeneration?

5. What is the connective tissue wrapping around a muscle that is continuous with tendons?

6. What is the lever system of the wrist?

7. What muscles would allow you to lift a weight?

   _____
   _____
   _____
   _____

8. What are the muscles that are used for fine control of the hand and fingers?

   _____
   _____
   _____
   _____

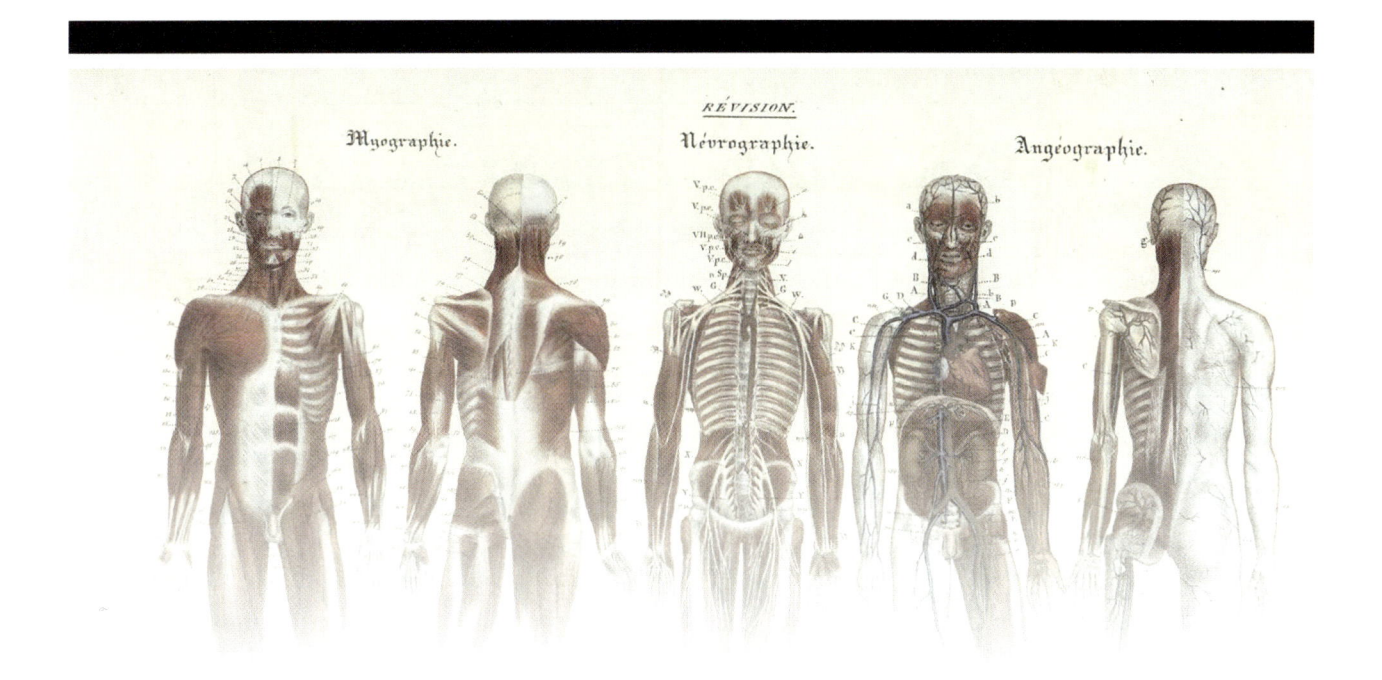

LOWER EXTREMITIES

Observation of Lower Limb Surface Anatomy and Procedure

PREPARATION

Before you begin to examine the surface anatomy of the lower limb, review the bone markings of the pelvis, femur, and tibia/fibula. Keep an articulated skeleton nearby during your observations to assist in the identification of bony landmarks and points of muscle attachment as you proceed. Alternatively, you can use the diagrams and illustrations in your book as a guide.

Identify on your laboratory partner, through visual observation and palpation, the surface anatomy of the lower limb, using the lab textbook for reference. For you to observe the surface anatomy in this region, your partner must be standing. Applying tension to the thigh and leg muscles will give greater definition to some muscles, improving your ability to observe them. Estimate the location of the structure, and then locate it specifically with visual observation and palpation.

The inferior width of the pelvis extends between the greater trochanters of the femurs. The lumbar vertebrae and median sacral crest of the sacrum are palpable just superior to the fold of buttock.

In the thigh, the sartorius muscle crosses the thigh diagonally from outside the hip (laterally) to the inner knee (medially), while the tensor fasciae latae forms a tight band, the iliotibial tract, on the lateral side of the thigh. The area of the femoral triangle is formed by three structures: (1) superiorly, by the inguinal ligament; (2) laterally, by the medial border of the sartorius muscle; and (3) medially, by the medial border of the adductor longus muscle. The femoral triangle is an important clinical site for obtaining blood samples or performing vascular catherization procedures.

Dissection of the Thigh

Muscles that Move the Thigh: Gluteal Muscles, Lateral Rotators of the Leg, Adductor Group, and Iliopsoas Group

To Be Observed On the Posterior Surface of the Thigh:

1. With the cadaver in the prone position, the muscles that rotate the thigh can be examined.
2. Begin your observation at the gluteal region or buttock.
3. The gluteal muscles can be observed to fill most of the gluteal surface and insert in various directions onto the femur.
4. Identify the gluteus maximus muscle and trace its fibers to the borders as it arises from the lumbodorsal fascia, sacrum, and iliac crest.
5. The iliac crest represents its most superior border.
6. The maximus is the largest extender and lateral rotator of the thigh.
7. Reflect the maximus (cut at the belly into medial and lateral portions) to expose underlying muscles and structures.
8. Observe the gluteus medius muscle deep and superior to the maximus and note the oblique angle at which the fibers run.
9. Deep to the belly of the medius lies the gluteus minimus muscle.
10. The minumus muscle abducts and medially rotates the thigh, but the medius only abducts.
11. The piriformis muscle is easily observed as it overlies the minimus just inferior to the medius, running horizontally from sacrum to greater trochanter of the femur.
12. Inferior to the piriformis is the small, somewhat triangular, tendon of the obturator internus muscle, which arises on the internal surface of the obturator foramen to insert on the medial surface of the greater trochanter of the femur.
13. The piriformis and obturator are lateral rotators of the thigh.
14. Identify on the lateral surface of the thigh the tensor fasciae latae muscle.
15. The tensor lies anterior and lateral to the gluteus medius and arises from the anterior superior iliac spine and crest.
16. Observe how the fibers of the tensor merge with those of the gluteus maximus, with both muscles inserting into the iliotibial tract.
17. Several layers of tough dense fascia form the iliotibial tract, which runs vertically down the lateral thigh therminating just inferior to the lateral epicondyle of the tibia.
18. The tract appears as a wide side stripe, like the stripe on tuxedo trousers.

To Be Observed On the Medial and Anterior Surfaces of the Thigh:

1. With the cadaver in the supine position, the adductor and flexor muscles of the thigh can be examined.
2. Identify the gracilis muscle, a long, belt-like muscle that runs vertically along the medial surface of the thigh.
3. It arises from the inferior rami of pubis and ischium to insert on the medial surface of the tibia.
4. At the medial border of the femoral triangle, identify the wedge-shaped pectineus muscle, which arises from the superior border of the pubis.
5. Between the pectimeus and gracilis muscles lies the adductor longus muscle.
6. Reflect the adductor longus to identify the adductor brevis muscle.
7. Reflect the adductor longus and the adductor brevius in order to identify the adductor magnus muscle.
8. This muscle lies deep to the longus and lateral to the gracilis and is the largest adductor muscle.
9. The iliopsoas is a muscle of the groin and is formed at its origin inside the pelvis by two separate muscles, the iliacus muscle and psoas muscle.
10. These muscles are clearly visible within the abdomen.
11. The iliacus muscle can be observed easily in the thigh just medial to the sartorius and deep to the femoral nerve.
12. The femoral triangle is an area formed by three sides, a floor, and a roof: (1) at the superior side by the boundry of the inguinal ligament; (2) laterally, by the medial border of the sartorius muscle; (3) medially, by the lateral border of the adductor longus muscle; (4) the roof or anterior wall is formed by the fascia lata; and (5) the floor por posterior wall is formed by the adductor longus, pectineus, and iliopsoas muscles.
13. Observe within the femoral triangle the femoral nerve, femoral artery, and femoral vein.
14. Begin your identification at the femoral nerve and proceed medially to identify the femoral artery and vein.

MUSCLES THAT MOVE THE LEG FLEXORS AND EXTENSORS

The muscles that move the leg originate on the thigh. The flexor muscles of the leg are located on the posterior surface of the femur, with the exception of the sartorius muscle. The sartorius muscle originates on the anterior surface of the pelvis. The knee extensor muscles are collectively referred to as the quadriceps femoris. The extensor group is composed of the vastus lateralis, vastus medialis, rectus femoris, and the vastus intermedius. All four of these muscles insert on the tibia through the patellar ligament.

To Be Observed On the Anterior Surface of the Thigh:

1. With the cadaver in the supine position, the extensors of the knee can be observed.
2. The four knee extensor muscles collectively known as the quadriceps femoris make up the bulk of the anterior thigh.
3. These muscles show up as distinct masses superior to the patella as the muscles collectively merge to insert into the patellar ligament.
4. Observe the rectus femoris muscle as it runs vertically in the center of the thigh.

5. The majority of the muscle can be traced from the anterior inferior iliac spine to insert on the tibial tuberosity via the patellar ligament.
6. Medially to the rectus, identify the vastus medialis muscle, which arises on the entire length of the linea aspera lateralis muscle, which arises inferior to the greater trochanter along the linea aspera and inserts the same as the rectus femoris.
7. Deep to the rectus femoris lies the fourth extensor of the leg, the vastus intermedius muscle.
8. Reflect the rectus femoris and observe the intermedius between the vastus medialis and lateralis muscles.
9. Identify the long belt-like sartorius muscle, which runs inferiorly at an oblique angle from the anterior superior iliac spine, medially to the medial surface of the tibia.
10. The sartorius is a flexor and lateral rotator of the thigh and not an extensor muscle.

To Be Observed On the Posterior Surface of the Thigh:

1. With the cadaver in the prone position, the muscles that flex the knee can be examined.
2. The semimembranosus, semitendinosus, and biceps femoris collectively make up the hamstring muscles.
3. The hamstrings are discernible as separate flexor muscles on the posterior and medial surfaces of the thigh.
4. These muscles simultaneously extend the hip and flex the knee, actions that occur together in walking.
5. Collectively, the hamstrings originate on the ischial tuberosity and linea aspera of the femur, and insert around the tibia and fibula.
6. By inserting around the knee, these muscles form a tripod and act as a knee stabilizer.
7. Identify first the wide flat semimembranosus muscle as it descends on the posteriomedial surface of the thigh.
8. From the adductor magnus trace the semimembranosus as it descends to the medial condule of the tibia.
9. Now observe the cylindrical semitendinosus muscle as it lies over the semimembranosus muscle and descends in the middle of the posterior thigh.
10. Reflect the gluteus maximus to observe the superior end of this muscle.
11. Trace the semitendinousus inferiorly and note how its tendon inserts on the posteromedial surface of the tibia.
12. The biceps femoris muscle lies somewhat parallel to these muscles as it descends on the posterolateral surface of the thigh.
13. This muscle has two origins, a long head and a short head.
14. The tendon of biceps femoris passes over the knee to insert laterally and anteriorly on the head of the fibula.

To Be Observed On the Posterior Surface of the Thigh (EXTRA)

Superior to the popliteal fossa, the sciatic nerve divides into a tibial nerve and a common fibular nerve. The tibial nerve can easily be observed deep to and between the biceps femoris and semitendinosus muscles. The femoral artery and vein continue into the leg respectively and the popliteal artery and popliteal vein are easily observed at this location. Parallel and slightly deep to the tibial nerve lies the popliteal vein; medial and parallel to the vein lies the popliteal artery. These nerves and blood vessels pass through the popliteal fossa into the leg.

To understand the relation between muscles, blood vessels, and nerves it is helpful to view these structures in transverse section. If a transverse section of the thigh is available for viewing, these relations can easily be observed.

LOCATE

The Pelvis and Lower Limb (from Anterior)
__ Inguinal ligament
__ Area of femoral triangle, site for palpation of femoral artery/vein
__ Tensor fasciae latae muscle
__ Sartorius muscle
__ Rectus femoris muscle
__ Vastus lateralis muscle
__ Vastus medialis muscle
__ Adductor longus muscle
__ Gracilis muscle
__ Patella
__ Tibial tuberosity

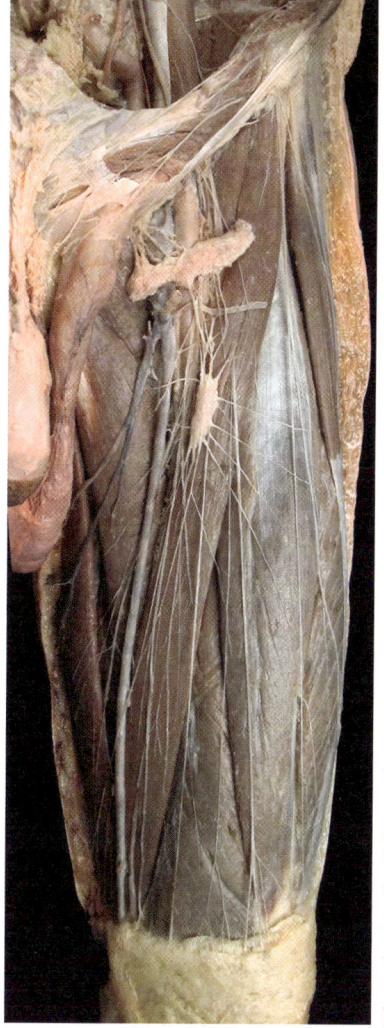

INFERIOR LIMB MODULE

The hamstring muscles are discernible as separate muscles on the posterior of the thigh. The vastus lateralis, rectus femoris, and vastus medialis muscles show up as distinct masses superior to the patella as the muscles merge into the patellar ligament. As you view the lower extremity from the posterior, the concave pit formed at the posterior side of the knee, the popliteal fossa, is delineated superiorly by the tendons of biceps femoris, semimembranosus, and semitendinosus muscles (hamstring muscles) and inferiorly by the medial and lateral heads of the gastrocnemius muscle. The gluteal muscles show quite well with the gluteus medius muscle appearing superior to the greater trochanter of the femur and the inferior border of the gluteus maximus muscle appearing as the fold of buttock.

Typically, the muscles of the leg show quite well. As you view the leg from the anterior, the anterior tibialis muscle is visible immediately to the lateral side of the tibial crest, the tendon of extensor digitorum longus is immediately lateral to that, and the fibularis longus muscle is lateral to the extensor digitorum longus. On the anterior surface of the tibia, the tibial tuberosity can be palpated where the quadriceps inserts. On the posterior side of the lower leg, the calf exhibits the medial and lateral heads of the gastrocnemius. The muscles are best displayed with your partner standing with both feet on tiptoe.

Lower Extremities

The Pelvis and Lower Limb (from Lateral)

__ Tensor fasciae latae muscle
               <Medius
__ Gluteus muscles <Maximus
__ Iliotibial tract
__ Vastus lateralis muscle
__ Semitendinous and semimembranosus muscle
__ Tendon of biceps femoris muscle
__ Popliteal fossa
__ Gastrocnemius muscle
__ Soleus muscle
__ Head of fibula
__ Patella
__ Patellar ligament
__ Tibial tuberosity
__ Fibularis longus muscle

The Pelvis and Lower Limb (from Posterior)

__ Iliac crest
__ Median sacral crest
               <Medius
__ Gluteus muscles<Maximus
__ Greater trochanter of femur
__ Location of sciatic nerve
__ Fold of buttock

__ Hamstring muscle group
__ Popliteal fossa
__ Tendon of biceps femoris muscle
__ Tendon of semitendinous muscle
__ Site for palpation of popliteal artery

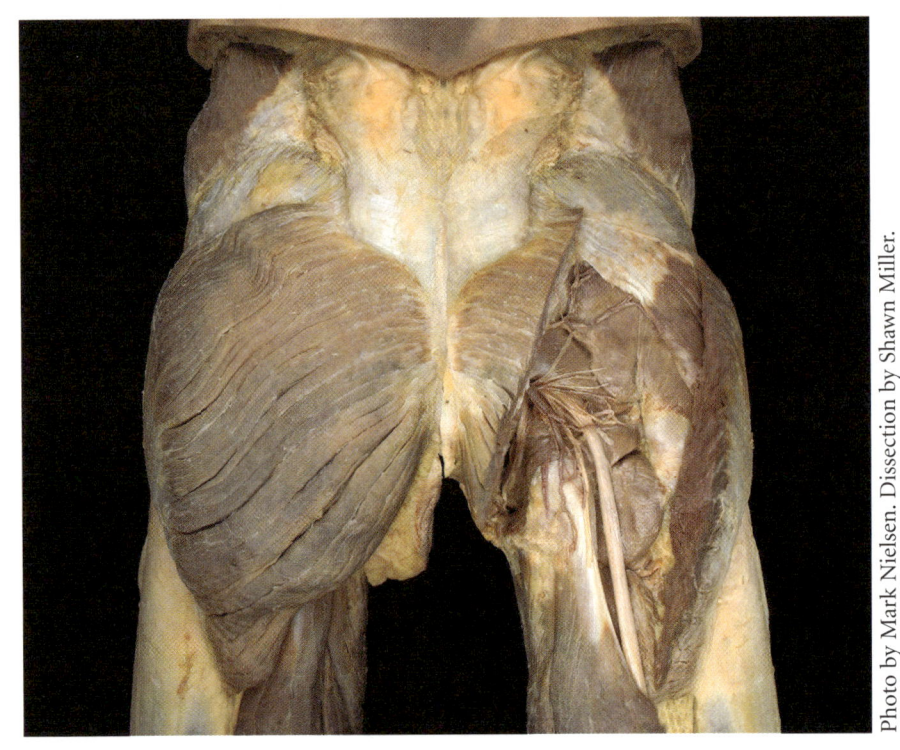

INFERIOR LIMB MODULE

Photo by Mark Nielsen. Dissection by Shawn Miller.

TABLE 6 *Muscles That Move the Thigh*

Muscle	Origin	Insertion	Action	Innervation
Gluteal Group				
Gluteus Maximus	Iliac crest of ilium, sacrum, coccyx, and lumbodorsal fascia	Iliotibial tract and gluteal tuberosity of femur	Extends and laterally rotates thigh	Inferior gluteal nerve
Gluteus Medius	Anterior iliac crest of ilium, lateral surface Between posterior and anterior gluteal lines	Greater trochanter of femur	Abducts and medially rotates thigh	Superior gluteal nerve
Gluteus Minimus	Lateral surface of ilium between inferior and anterior gluteal lines	Greater trochanter of femur	Abducts and medially rotates thigh	As above
Tensor Fascia lata	Iliac crest and lateral surface of anterior Superior iliac spine	Iliotibial tract	Flexes, abducts and medially rotates thigh; tenses fascia lata, which laterally supports the knee	As above
Lateral Rotator Group				
Obturators (externus and internus) foramen	Lateral and medial margins of obturator	Trochanteric fossa of femur (externus); medial surface of greater trochanter (internus)	Laterally rotates thigh	Obturator nerve (externus) and special nerve from sacral plexus (internus)
Piriformis	Anterolateral surface of sacrum	Greater trochanter of femur	Laterally rotates and abducts thigh	Branches of sacral nerves
Gemelli (superior and inferior)	Ischial spine and tuberosity	Medial surface of greater trochanter	Laterally rotates thigh	Nerves to obturator internus and quadratus femoris
Quadratus femoris	Lateral border of ishial tuberosity	Intertrochanteric crest of femur	Laterally rotates thigh	Special nerve from sacral plexus
Adductor Group				
Adductor brevis	Inferior ramus of pubis	Linea aspera of femur	Adducts, medially rotates, and flexes thigh	Obturator nerve
Adductor longus	Inferior ramus of pubis anterior to brevis	As above	Adducts, flexes, and medially rotates thigh	As above

Lower Extremities

TABLE 6 *Muscles That Move the Thigh continued...*

Muscle	Origin	Insertion	Action	Innervation
Adductor magnus	Inferior ramus of pubis posterior to adductor brevis and ischial tuberosity	Linear aspera and adductor tubercle of femur	Adducts thigh; superior portion flexes, and medially rotates thigh, inferior portion extends and laterally rotates thigh	Obturator and sciatic nerves
Pectineus	Superior ramus of pubis	Pectineal line Inferior to lesser trochanter of femur	Flexes, medially rotates, and adducts thigh	Femoral nerve
Gracilis	Inferior ramus of pubis	Medial surface of tibia inferior to medial condyle	Flexes leg, adducts, and medially rotates thigh	Obturator nerve
Iliopsoas Group				
Iliacus	Iliac fossa of ilium	Femur distal to lesser trochanter; tendon fused with that of psoas	Flexes hip and/or lumber spine	Femoral nerve
Psoas major	Anterior surfaces and transverse processes of vertebrae T12-L5	Lesser trochanter in company with iliacus	As above	Branches of the lumbar plexus

Adductor Group (Anterior and Posterior Views)

__Adductor brevis
__Adductor longus
__Adductor magnus
__Pectineus
__Gracilis
              <Iliacus
__Iliopsoas group   <Psoas major

TABLE 7 *Muscles That Move the Leg*

Muscle	Origin	Insertion	Action	Innervation
Flexors of the Leg				
Biceps femoris	Ishial tuberosity and linea aspera of femur	Head of fibula, lateral condyle of tibia	Flexes leg, extends and laterally rotates thigh	Sciatic nerve; tibial portion (to long head) and common fibular branch (to short head)
Semimembranosus	Ischial tuberosity	Posterior surface of medial condyle of tibia	Flexes and medially rotates leg, extends thigh	Sciatic nerve (tibial portion)
Semitendinosus	Ischial tuberosity	Proximal, medial surface of tibia near insertion of gracilis	As above	As above
Sartorius	Anterior superior iliac spine	Medial surface of tibia near tibial tuberosity	Flexes leg, flexes and laterally rotates thigh	Femoral nerve
Popliteus	Lateral condyle of femur	Posterior surface of proximal tibial shaft	Medially rotates tibia (or laterally rotates femur)	Tibial nerve
Extensors of the Leg				
Rectus femoris	Anterior inferior iliac spine and superior acetabular rim of ilium	Tibial tuberosity via patellar ligement	Extends leg, flexes thigh	Femoral nerve
Vastus intermedius	Anterolateral surface of femur and linea aspera (distal half)	As above	Extends leg	As above
Vastus lateralis	Anterior and Inferior to greater trochanter of femur and along linea aspera (proximal half)	As above	As above	As above
Vastus medialis	Entire length of linea aspera of femur	As above	As above	As above

Dissection of Lower Extremities

> **Required Instruments**
> Scalpel   Blade size 22   Saw   Blade size 10   Retractors   Handles 3,4

Dissection of the Anterior Thigh

1. With the cadaver in supine position, expose the anterior thigh muscles by carefully removing the superficial fascia.
2. Identify the longer muscle of the thigh, the sartorius, and the margin of the inguinal ligament. On the lateral, identify the adductor longus.
3. By carefully incising along the fascia lata, you are able to expose the femoral triangle, which contains the femoral artery, femoral vein, and femoral nerve.
4. Continue your dissection to identify and expose the deep femoral artery and its branches.
5. Turn your attention to the major anterior thigh muscles, which are the rectus femoris muscle and the vastus lateralis and vastus medialis.
6. You may make an incision on the quadriceps femoris tendon to reflect it superiorly and expose the vastus intermedialis muscle.
7. Observe the extension of the quadriceps femoris tendon over the patella and its insertion of the tibial tuberosity.

Dissection of the Medial Thigh

1. Observe that the muscles on the medial side of the thigh are adductors.
2. Expose the gracilis muscle with the blunt dissection.
3. The pectineus muscle can be separated by blunt dissection.
4. Continue blunt dissection to identify and isolate the adductor brevis and the adductor longus muscles.
5. Continue to identify and follow the trail of the obturator nerve as it emerges from the obturator foramen and supplies the external obturator muscle and the adductor muscles.
6. Identify the adductor magnum, as it is a more prominent muscle among the adductor group.
7. Note the entrance of the femoral artery and femoral vein into the adductor hiatus.

LOCATE

Gluteal Muscle Group (Posterior and Lateral Views)

__Gluteal group
                    <Gluteus maximus
                    <Gluteus medius
                    <Gluteus minimus

__Tensor fasciae latae
__Iliotibial tract (band)

Lateral Rotator Group (Anterior and Posterior Views)

__Obturators (internal and external)   __Piriformis

Dissection of the Posterior Thigh

1. As the skin of the cadaver has been removed, continue dissection with the cadaver in the prone position.
2. After exposing the iliotibial trail by removing the overlying tissue, separate the fascial lata from the underlying flexor muscles of the thigh.
3. Observe the origin of the fascia lata muscle at the iliac crest.
4. Preserving the sacrotuberous ligament, incise the origin of the gluteus maximus muscle at the inferior border.
5. Incise and deflect the piriformis muscle to expose the underlying sciatic nerve, which is thicker and more prominent compared to the posterior femoral cutaneoys nerve of the thigh.
6. Continue the dissection to expose the superior and inferior gluteal nerves and arteries.
7. When the gluteus medius is divided and deflected, you can expose the gluteus minimus muscle.
8. Continue dissection along the same margin to expose the tendons of the superior and inferior glumellus muscles and the internal obturator muscles at their insertion.
9. Inferior to the gemellus muscles, the quadratus femoris muscle can be exposed as part of the rotator group.
10. The tendon of the external obturator muscle can be exposed by dissecting deep into the lateral rotator group.
11. This dissection is more effective if you periodically rotate the leg at the hip joint to observe the interrelationship of these muscles.
12. The posterior thigh muscles of the hamstring group can be isolated by blunt dissection.
13. These hamstring muscles originate at the ischial tuberosity and you can continue the dissection along their length to the sacrotuberous ligament.
14. The short and long heads of the biceps femoris muscle can be separated along with the semitendinous and the semimembranous muscles.
15. Continue the dissection to identify the underlying adductor magnus muscle.
16. Along the same muscle you can also observe the sciatic nerve extending to the popliteal fossa.
17. The sciatic nerve divides into the tibial nerve and the common peroneal (fibular) nerve at the popliteal fossa.

18. Continue the dissection to expose the popliteal artery and vein.
19. With gentle manipulation, identify the margins of the hip joint and incise the capsule of the hip joint.
20. When the capsule has been adequately incised, the head of the femur and the acetabular cavity will be distinctly exposed.
21. At the head of the femur is the ligamentum teres, which attaches deep into the acetabular fossa.
22. Observe the acetabular cavity, its margins, and its articular cartilage.
23. Observe erosion of the cartilage, which corresponds with the cadaver's age.

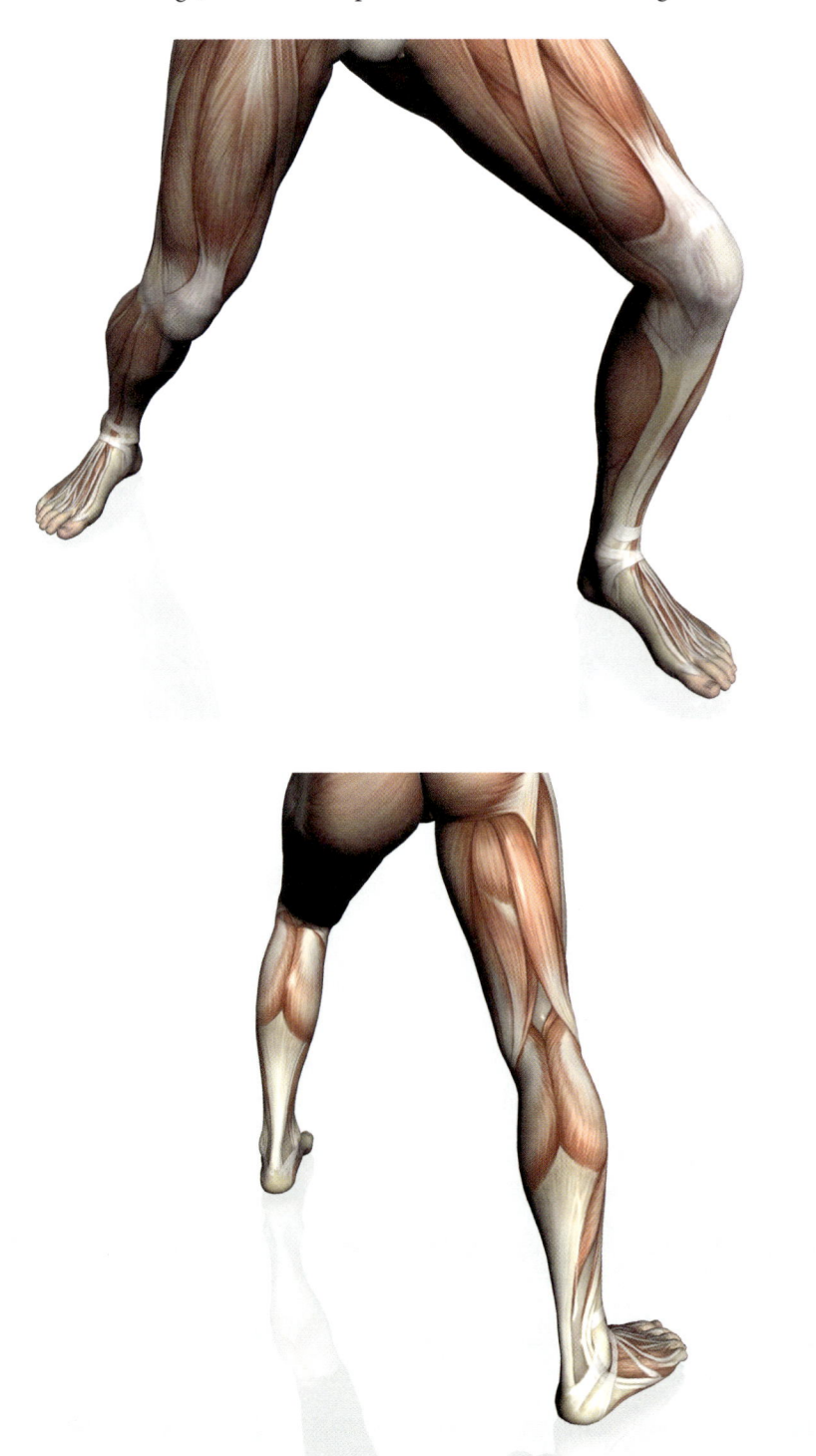

LOCATE

Extensors of the Leg (Anterior View)

     <Rectus Femoris
__Quadriceps <Vastus intermedius
     <Vastus lateralis
     <Vastus medialis
__Sartorius (flexor)

Flexors of the Leg (Posterior View)

__Biceps femoris   __Sartorius
__Semimembranous   __Popliteal
__Semitendinous

To Be Observed On the Posterior Leg (Calf)

With the cadaver in the prone position, the muscles that move the foot and toes can be examined. The superficial leg muscles—the gastrocnemius, soleus, and popliteus—will be observed first. Return to the popliteal fossa and at the inferior border of this area, identify the medial and lateral heads of the gastrocnemius muscle. The heads originate respectively from just superior to the medial and lateral condyles of the femur. Trace the gastrocnemius inferiorly and observe how its fibers insert into the calcaneal tendon or Achilles tendon. The massive calcaneal tendon inserts on the posterior surface of the calcaneus bone. Deep to the gastrocnemius lies the thin, broad flat soleus muscle. The soleus arises from the head of the fibula and the posteromedial shaft of the tibia and is totally covered by the gastrocnemius; only its medial and lateral borders are exposed. Reflect the medial and lateral heads of the gastrocnemius (cut at their orgins) and observe the soleus. Notice the soleus and gastrocnemius share a common tendon, the calcaneal tendon. The soleus muscle and both heads of the gastrocnemius form the muscular mass of the calf. On the medial surface of the gastrocnemius, the saphenous nerve and great saphenous vien may be observed.

The small, slightly triangular popliteus muscle arises from the lateral femoral condyle within the fibrous capsule of the knee joint, crosses the knee joint at an oblique angle, from lateral to medial, to insert onto the proximal posterior surface of the tibia. Observe the popliteus deep to the lateral head of the gastrocnemius (reflected) within the popliteal fossa. The action of the popliteus is to rotate medially the tibia. The knee joint is locked during extension simply because there is more travel on the medial condyle than on the lateral condyle, which accounts for medial rotation of the femur on the tibia.

To Be Observed On the Medial Surface of the Leg

The deep calf muscles are primarily concerned with plantar flexion of the foot and flexion of the toes and send their tendons across the ankle into the foot. These muscles are best observed by reflecting the gastrocnemius and soleus. Keep these muscles reflected as you observe the deep muscles from medial to lateral sides of the leg. Begin on the medial side and identify the flexor digitorum longus. Trace its tendon as it passes just posterior to the medial malleolus at the ankle and under the extenson retinaculum, inserting on the inferior surfaces of toes 2-5. Now identify the tibialis posterious, which lies immediately lateral and runs parallel to the flexor digitorum longus. Trace its tendon and note that it runs a course similar to the flexor, but inserts at numerous points on the plantar surface of the foot. The tibial nerve may be observed on the surface of the tibialis posterior. Identify the flexor hallucis longus as it lies on the posterior surface of the fibula, just lateral to the tibialis posterior. Trace the tendon on the flexor hallucis longus and note that it runs posterior to the other muscles, inserting on the inferior surface of the distal phalanx of the great toe.

To Be Observed On the Anterior and Lateral Surfaces of the Leg

With the cadaver in the supine position the muscles that move the foot and toes can be examined. The anterior of the leg has very little musculature. Tendons of the muscles that move the foot and toes must cross the ankle and pass deep to the retinacula. Identify on the anterior surface of these tendons, just superior to the ankle, the connective tissue fibers of the superior extensor retinaculum. Just inferior the the ankle identify the inferior extenson retinaculum as it arises from the lateral surface of the calcaneus and passes superiorly to overlie the tendons of the extensor digitorum longus and extensor hallucis longus.

On the anterolateral side of the leg identify the large tibialis anterior muscle as it runs inferiorly and parallel to the lateral surface of the tibial shaft. Trace the muscle and observe how it arises from the shaft and interosseous membrane to form a large tendon that crosses the anterior surface of the ankle. The tendon passes medially deep to the superior and inferior extensor retinacula to insert on the base of the first metatarsal.

The superficial extensor hallucis longus muscle lies lateral and somewhat deep to the tibialis anterior. Reflect the tibialis anterior medially and observe the extensor as it arises from the anterior medial surface of the fibula, then trace its tendon inferiorly. The extensor digitorum longus is best identified just lateral to the tendon of the tibialis anterior. Trace the muscle superiorly to the lateral condyle of the tibia. Now trace the muscle inferiorly and observe its tendon. The extensor tendons cross the ankle to pass deep to the superior and inferior extenson retinacula. The tendon of the extensor digitorum longus divides into four tendons to insert on the dorsal surfaces of toes 2-5.

Identify on the lateral surface of the leg the superficial fibularis longus muscle. Trace this muscle from the lateral condyle of the tibia to its tendon, which crosses the ankle posterior to the lateral malleolus to then pass under the inferior peroneal retinaculum to the base of the first metatarsal. Superior to the ankle the bulk of the fibularis brevis muscle can be identified under the tendon of the longus. The tendon of the brevis follows the same course but inserts on the base of the fifth metatarsal. The common fibular nerve can be observed between the peroneus muscles near the neck of the fibula.

To understand the relation between muscles, blood vessels, and nerves it is helpful to view the leg structures in transverse section.

LOCATE

Superficial Muscles (Posterior Surface of the Leg)
__Gastrocnemius (medial and lateral heads)
__Soleus
__Calcaneal (Achilles) tendon
__Popliteal

Deep Muscles (Posterior Surface of the Leg)
__Fibularis longus
__Fibularis brevis
__Flexor hallucis longus
__Tibialis posterior
__Flexor digitorum longus
__Tendon of fibularis brevis
__Tendon of fibularis longus

Superficial Muscles of the Leg (Lateral View)

__Tibialis anterior
__Fibularis longus
__Fibularis brevis
__Extensor digitorum longus
__Soleus
__Lateral head of gastrocnemius
__Calcaneal tendon
__Inferior extensor retinaculum

Superficial Muscles of the Leg (Medial View)

__Patellar tendon (ligament)
__Tibialis anterior
__Soleus
__Gastrocnemius
__Calcaneal tendon
__Tendon of tibialis anterior

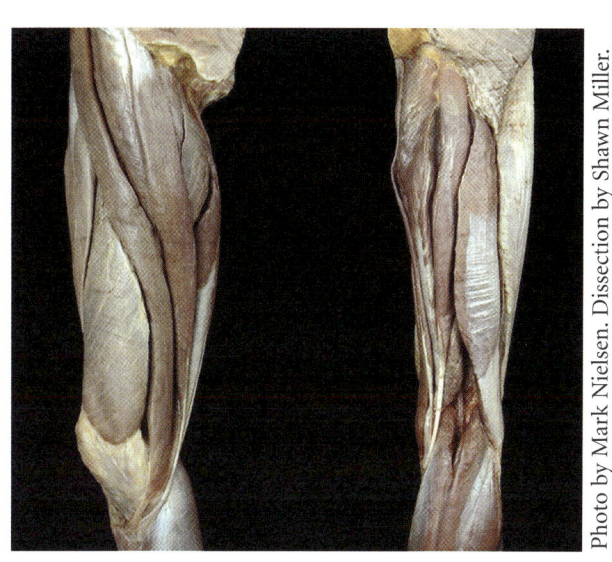

INFEROR LIMB MODULE

Anterior Surface (Lower Leg)

__Patellar tendon (ligament)
__Fibularis longus
__Tibialis anterior
__Extensor digitorum longus
__Extensor hallucis longus
__Superior extensor retinaculum
__Inferior extensor retinaculum

Dissection of the Leg

Required Instruments
Scalpel   Blade size 22   Saw   Blade size 10   Retractors   Handles 3,4

1. Make an incision that extends from the suprapatellar margin to the ankle.

2. Continue dissection of the skin medially and laterally to expose the muscle of the anterior leg.

3. Identify and subsequently separate the four muscles that comprise the anterior compartment.

4. Identify and separate the anterior tibialis muscle and continue to separate the extensor digitorum longus and the extensor hallucis longus including the fibularis tertius.

5. On the lateral aspect, identify and separate the muscles along the fibula, the fibularis longus, and the fibularis brevis. These muscles constitute the lateral compartment.

6. Continue dissecting the skin over the dorsum of the foot extending it from the ankle to the toes.

7. This will expose the tendons of the muscles, especially the extensor digitorum under the superior and inferior extensor retinaculum.

8. After exposing the fibularis muscles, identify the peroneal /fibular nerve.

9. Turn your attention to the posterior aspect of the leg and expose the muscles compressing the posterior compartment.

10. Start by extending the dissection of the skin over the posterior surface of the compartment, the gastrocnemius.

11. Along with the gastrocnemius, identify and separate the soleus.

12. Continue identifying and separating the posterior tibialis muscle and the plantaris, popliteal along with the flexor muscles of the toes and the great toe, which are the flexor digitorum.

13. Longus and that of the great toe, the flexor hullucis longus.

    *All these seven muscles constitute the posterior compartment.

14. You may incise the two heads of the gastrocnemius and reflect it for better exposure of the soleus.

15. By carefully reflecting the soleus, the tibial nerve can be exposed.

16. This dissection will expose the posterior tibial artery and its branch to the fibular side, the fibular artery.

17. Posterior to the medial malleolus, you can observe the tendons of the flexor digitorum longus, the flexor hallucis longus, and of the tibialis posterior.

MUSCLES THAT MOVE THE FOOT AND TOES

The muscles that move the foot and toes take part in the act of walking. The muscles of the calf, gastrocnemius and soleus, allow for plantar flexion. These muscles share a single tendon, the calcaneal tendon, or Achilles tendon. The muscles that move the toes originate on the tibia, fibula, or both. The tendons of these muscles cross the ankle joint deep to stabilize the connective sheath bands, the superior extensor retinaculum, inferior extensor retinaculum, and flexor retinaculum. This arrangement of muscles is similar to those that move the hand.

Procedure

Before you begin to examine the muscles that move the foot and toes, review the bone markings of the distal ends of the tibia and fibula and ankle and bones of the foot. Keep an articulated skeleton nearby to aid you in identifying bony landmarks and points of muscle attachment as you proceed.

Identify the following **leg muscles, skeletal elements,** and **associated structures**, using a leg torso model or prosected cadaver specimen. The origin, insertions, and actions of the muscles that move the foot and toes are presented in Table 8, and should be reviewed and referred to as you proceed in your observation. Observe these muscles first on the model before proceeding to the cadaver.

LOCATE

Dorsal Surface

__Superior/inferior extensor retinaculum
__Extensor digitorum brevis
__Abductor hallucis
__Interossei dorsal (4)

Plantar View (Superficial and Deep Layers)

__Plantar aponeurosis
__Calcaneus
__Abductor hallucis
__Flexor digitorum brevis
__Flexor digiti minimi
__Abductor digiti minimi
__Quadratus plantae
__Lumbricals (4)
__Flexor hallucis brevis
__Adductor hallucis
__Interossei, dorsal (4)
__Inerossei, plantar (3)

OBSERVATION OF ANKLE AND FOOT

Identify on your laboratory partner........ADD MORE

LOCATE

Knee, Leg, Ankle, and Foot (from Anterior)

__ Patella
__ Tibial tuberosity
__ Gastrocnemius muscle
__ Soleus muscle
__ Fibularis longus muscle
__ Anterior border of tibia
__ Tibialis anterior muscle
__ Medial malleolus
__ Great saphenous vein
__ Lateral malleolus
__ Tendon of extensor hallucis longus muscle
__ Tendons of extensor digitorum longus muscle
__ Dorsal venous arch

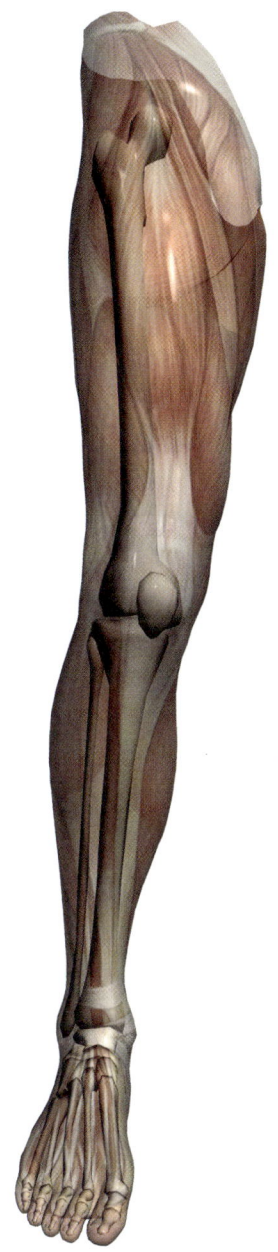

ANTERIOR KNEE LEG

© Patrick Hermans, 2010. Used under license from Shutterstock, Inc.

Lower Extremities

Knee, Leg, Ankle, and Foot (from Posterior)

__ Site for palpation of popliteal artery
__ Site for palpation of common peroneal nerve
                                     <Lateral
__ Gastrocnemius, muscle heads   <Media
__ Soleus
__ Calcaneal tendon
__ Tendon of fibularis longus muscle
__ Medial malleolus
__ Lateral malleolus
__ Site for palpation of posterior tibial artery
__ Calcaneus

Dissection of the Foot

Required Instruments
Scalpel   Blade size 22   Saw   Blade size 10
Retractors   Handles 3,4

1. Make a vertical incision on the skin extending from the ankle to the middle of the toes and a transverse incision along the border of the distal margin of the metatarsals.

2. Extend the dissection medially and laterally to expose the dorsal and plantar surfaces of the foot.

3. On the lateral side of the foot, dissect and separate the abductor digitalis minimus muscle.

4. On the medial aspect, dissect and separate the abductor hallucis muscle.

5. By further dissection, deep in the plantar surface, you can identify the flexor digitorum longus along with the lumbrical muscles.

6. From the tendon of the flexor digitorum, you can dissect and identify the plantar quadratus muscle.

7. The flexor hallucis longus muscle can be identified on the medial aspect of the foot.

8. Continue deeper dissection to expose the tendon of the flexor muscles: the flexor digitalis minimi and the flexor hallucis brevis.

9. Further exploration can help palpate the sesamoid bones of the foot.

10. Through deeper dissection, continue to identify the interosseus muscles on the plantar surface.

11. By gently moving the foot at the joint of the cadaver, closely observe the ligamentous structures surrounding it.

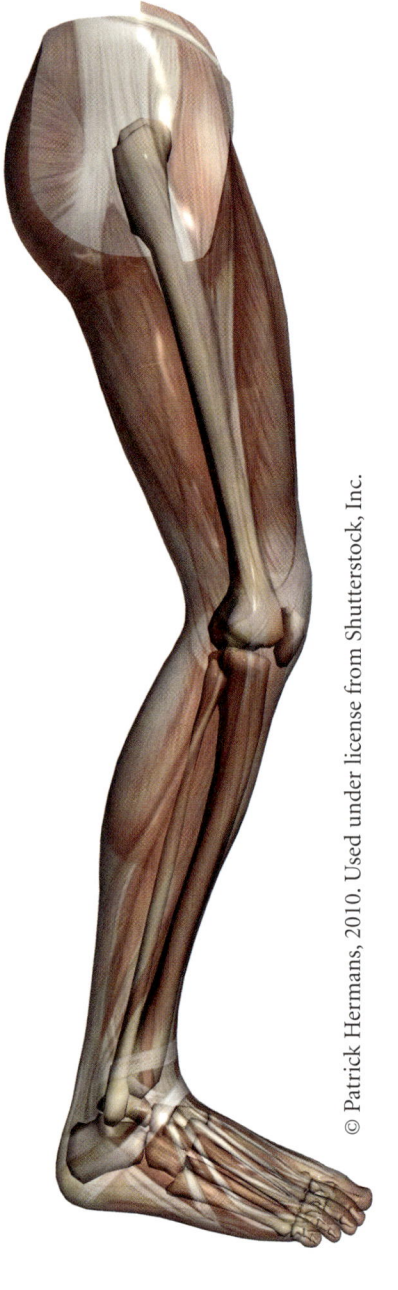

POSTERIOR KNEE LEG ANKLE FOOT

Name _____ Date _____

LOWER EXTREMITIES

Laboratory Review Questions

1. The muscles of the quadriceps femoris group insert where?

2. What are the flexors of the leg?

3. What is the common tendon shared by the gastrocnemius and the soleus muscles?

4. What is a common injection site that allows us to avoid the sciatic nerve?

5. What are the attachments for the medial thigh muscles?

6. The patella lies within the tendon of the _____, which inserts on the _____.

Lower Extremities 57

7. Describe a sesamoid bone.

8. What is the femoral triangle bound by?

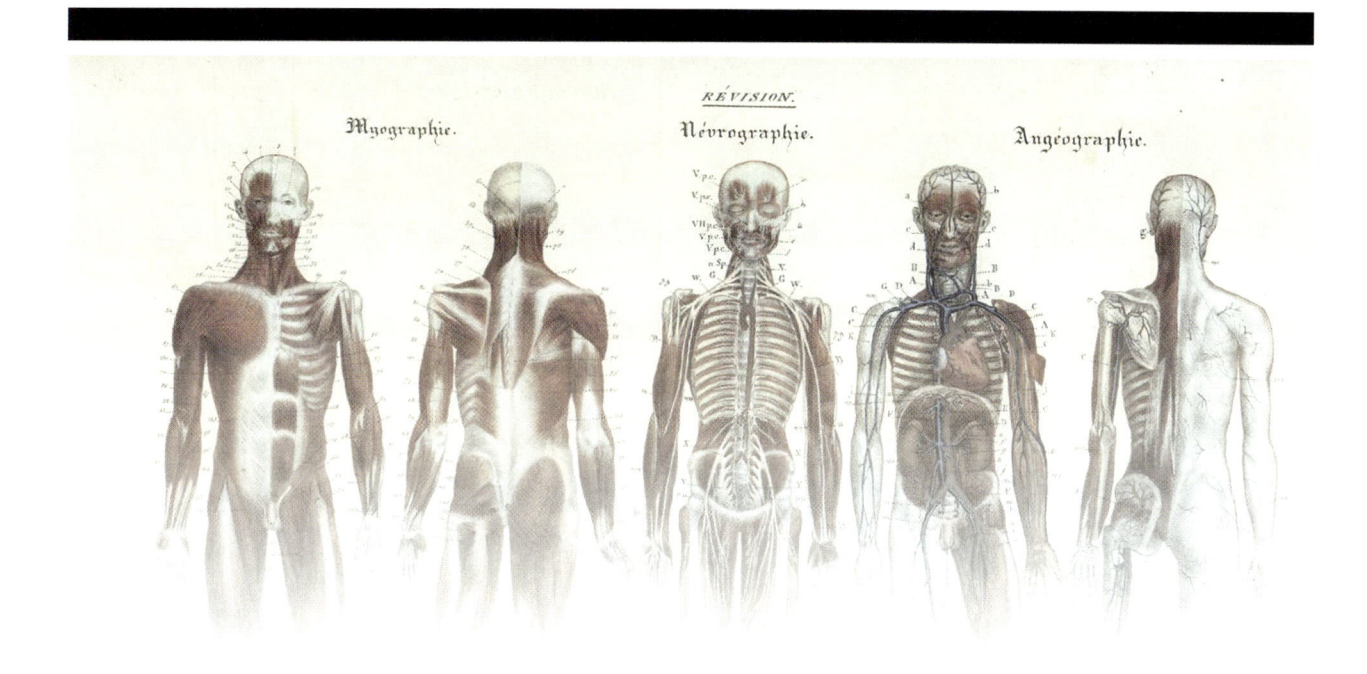

HEAD AND NECK REGION

Dissection of the Head and Neck Region

LOCATE

Head and Neck (from Anterior)

___Supraorbital margin
___Auricle (external ear)
___Zygomatic bone
___Body of mandible
___Mental protuberance
___Thyroid cartilage
___Cricoid cartilage

___Suprasternal notch
___Sternum (manubrium)
___Sternocleidomastoid muscle >Clavicle head
                                           >Sternal head
___Trapezius muscle
___Clavicle

Head and Neck (Posterior and Anterior Triangles)

___Angle of mandible
___Mastoid process
___Site for palpation of submandibular gland and submandibular lymph nodes
___Hyoid bone
___Site for palpation of pulse of facial artery

___Site for palpation of carotid pulse
___External jugular vein beneath platysma muscle
___Posterior triangle

___Origin of brachial plexus
___Clavicle

___Trapezius muscle
___Thyroid cartilage
___Supraclavicular fossa
___Anterior triangle
___Suprasternal notch

___Sternocleidomastoid >Clavicular head
   muscle   >Sternal head
___Acromion process

Dissection of the Head and Neck Region

Required Instruments
Scalpel   Blade size 22   Retractors   Handles 3,4

1. Make an incision of the skin covering the neck to the inferior margin of the mandible.
2. Start a longitudinal incision at the mental depression and extend it down to the manubrium.
3. Laterally extend the previous incision to the right and left along the inferior margin of the mandible.
4. Continue to dissect the skin and deflect it further to the right and the left to expose the neck.
5. Identify the thyroid cartilage superior to the thyroid gland.
6. Identify the two lobes of the thyroid gland right and left of the isthmus.
7. Identify the hyoid bone and observe the muscles and ligaments surrounding it.
8. Identify the platysma muscle and remove it from the neck to expose the external jugular vein along with the auricular and retromandibular veins.
9. Identify also the facial vein and the anterior jugular vein as they converge toward the external jugular vein.
10. Continue dissection to identify the sternocleidomastoid muscle from its origin at the sternum and clavicle and its insertion at the mastoid process.
11. Make an incision at the insertion of the sternocleidomastoid muscle and reflect it to expose the underlying vessels and nerves.
12. The common carotid artery and its bifurcation can be exposed after you dissect the carotid sheath.

Name _____ Date _____

HEAD AND NECK REGION
Laboratory Review Questions

1. What are the muscles of mastication?

2. What muscle is used to turn the head?

3. What is the function of the sinuses?

4. Where does the spinal cord enter the skull?

5. List the names of the sutures of the skull and which bones they attach.

6. What is another name for the "eye socket"?

7. When searching for human remains, which is the bone most likely to be missing from the skull and why?

   _____
   _____
   _____
   _____

8. By which joints are the teeth held into place?

   _____
   _____
   _____
   _____

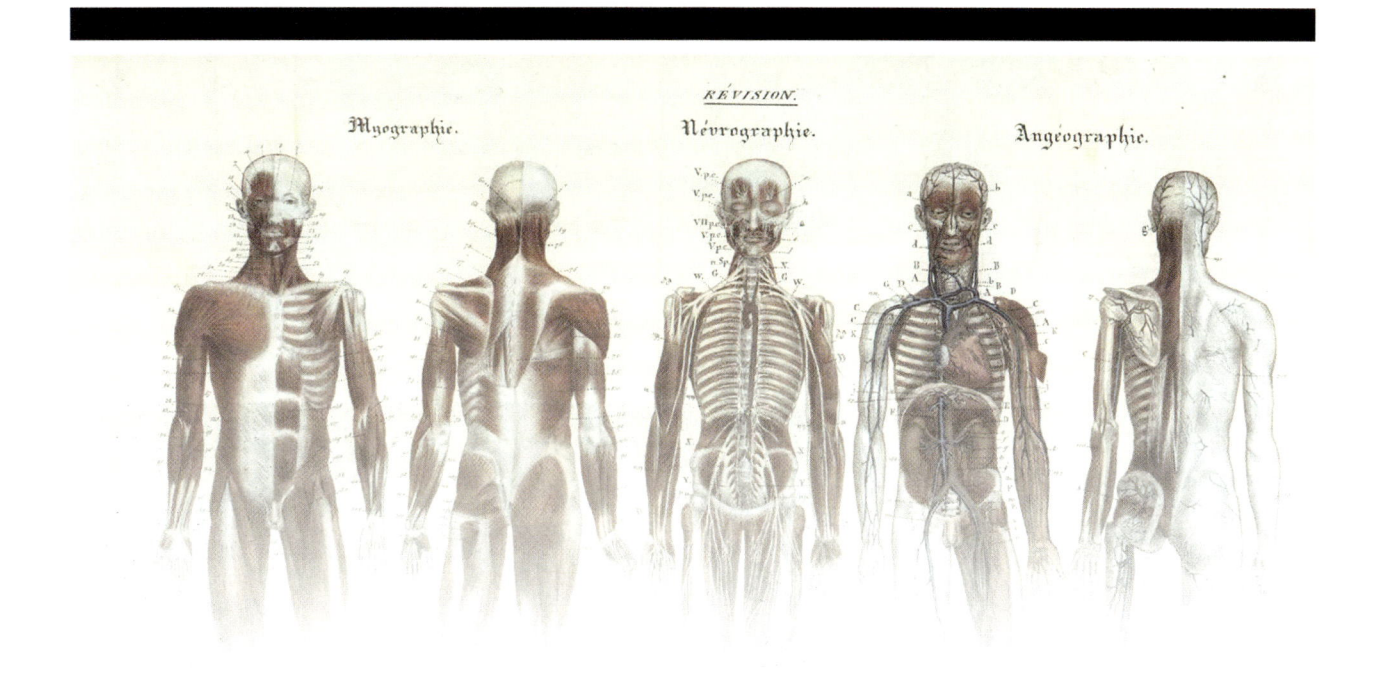

THE SKELETAL SYSTEM AND ARTICULATION

THE SKELETAL SYSTEM: Axial Division

OBSERVATION: THE AXIAL DIVISION, SKULL

Bones of the skull protect the brain and guard the entrances to the digestive and respiratory systems. The skull contains 22 bones: 8 form the cranium (braincase) and 14 form the face. Additionally, the hyoid bone and the auditory ossicles (3 within each ear), the mallet-shaped malleus, the anvil-shaped incus, and the stirrup-shaped stapes are associated with the skull. Use the mnemonic MIS for these bones. Bones of the skull are firmly attached together with ossified dense fibrous connective tissue to form immovable joints called sutures. The coronal, sagittal, squamosal, and lambdoid sutures are easily identified on the adult skull.

LOCATE

__ Frontal bone
__ Parietal bone
__ Occipital bone
__ Sphenoid bone
__ Temporal bones
__ Maxillary bones (maxilla)
__ Zygomatic bones
__ Mandible
__ Nasal bones
__ Lacrimal bones
__ Ethmoid

SUTURES: THE ADULT SKULL

LOCATE

__ Sagittal suture
__ Coronal suture
__ Squamosal suture
__ Lambdoid suture

THE ADULT SKULL

LOCATE

Posterior View

__ Sagittal suture
__ Parietal bone (paired bones)
__ Lambdoid suture
__ Occipital bone
__ External occipital protuberance
__ Occipital condyle
__ Squamous suture
__ Temporal bone (paired bone)
__ Mastoid process
__ Styloid process

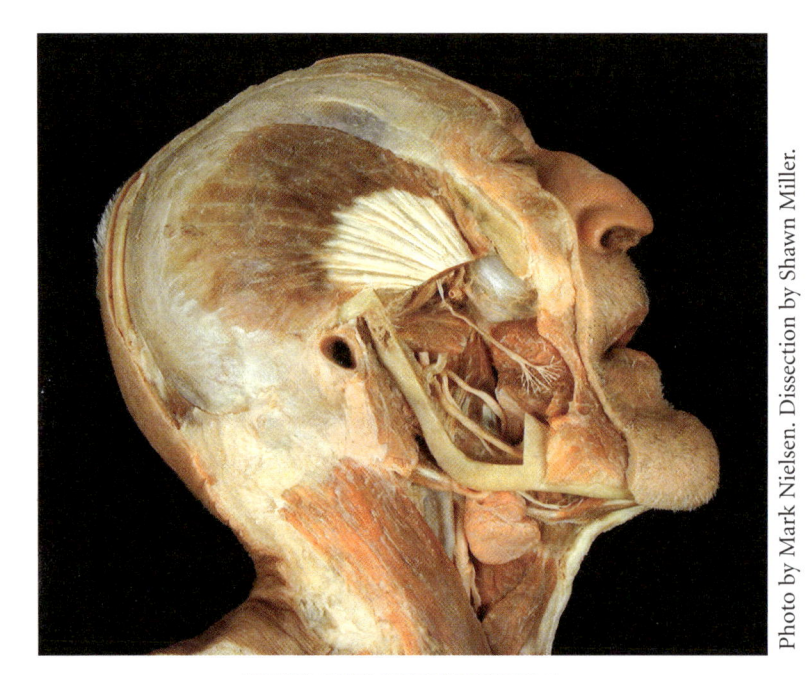

HEAD AND NECK MODULE

IDENTIFY AND LOCATE

Superior View

__ Sagittal suture
__ Parietal bone
__ Lambdoid bone
__ Occipital bone
__ Coronal bone
__ Frontal bone
__ Nasal bones
__ Zygomatic bones (paired bones)
__ Temporal bones

IDENTIFY AND LOCATE

Lateral View

__ Frontal bone
__ Coronal suture
__ Parietal bone
__ Superior temporal line
   (not clearly defined on all specimens)
__ Inferior temporal line
   (not clearly defined on all specimens)
__ Squamous suture
__ Lambdoid suture
__ Occipital bone
__ Supraorbital foramen
__ Temporal bone
__ External auditory meatus (canal)
__ Mastoid process
__ Styloid process

__ Zygomatic bone
                                                              <Zygomatic process
                                                              <of temporal bone
__ Zygomatic arch   <Temporal process
                                                              <of zygomatic bone
__ Sphenoid bone
__ Nasal bone
__ Lacrimal bone
__ Nasolacrimal groove of lacrimal bone
__ Ethmoid bone
__ Maxilla
__ Infraorbital foramen
__ Mandible
__ Mental foramen
__ Mental protuberance of mandible

IDENTIFY AND LOCATE

Anterior View

__ Coronal suture
__ Parietal bone
__ Frontal bone
__ Supraorbital foramen (or notch)
__ Temporal bone
__ Mastoid process
__ Zygomatic bone
__ Zygomaticofacial foramen
__ Temporal process of zygomatic bone
__ Ethmoid bone
__ Perpendicular plate of ethmoid bone

__ Vomer bone
__ Middle nasal concha
__ Inferior nasal concha
__ Lacrimal bone
__ Nasal bone
__ Frontonasal suture
__ Maxilla
__ Infraorbital foramen
__ Mandible
__ Mental protuberance of mandible
__ Mental foramen

IDENTIFY AND LOCATE

Inferior View

__ Occipital bone
__ External occipital protuberance
__ Superior nuchal line

__ Occipital condyle

__ Carotid canal
__ Foramen spinosum
__ Foramen lacerum
__ Foramen ovale
__ Mandibular fossa

- Fossa for cerebellum
- Occipitomastoid suture
- Lambdoid suture
- Stylomastoid foramen (mastoid foramen)
- Temporal bone
- Mastoid process
- Styloid process
- External auditory canal
- Jugular foramen
- Jugular fossa
- Maxilla
- Incisive fossa
- Horizontal plate of palatine bone
- Palatine foramen (greater and lesser)
- Sphenoid bone
- Pterygoid processes (medial and lateral)
- Vomer
- Zygomatic arch
- Zygomatic bone

SECTIONAL ANATOMY OF THE SKULL

IDENTIFY AND LOCATE

Horizontal Section

- Frontal bone
- Frontal sinus
- Ethmoid bone
- Crista galli
- Cribriform plate
- Sphenoid bone
- Sella turcica
- Optic canal (foramen)
- Foramen rotundum
- Foramen lacerum
- Foramen ovale
- Foramen spinosum
- Carotid canal
- Temporal bone
- Petrous portion of temporal bone
- Internal acoustic meatus
- Foramen magnum
- Jugular foramen
- Hypoglossal canal
- Parietal bone
- Occipital bone

Sagittal Section

- Frontal bone
- Frontal sinus
- Coronal suture
- Parietal bone
- Lambdoid suture
- Occipital bone
- Margin of foramen magnum
- Occipital condyle
- Temporal bone
- Styloid process
- Petrous portion of temporal bone
- Internal acoustic meatus
- Jugular foramen
- Hypoglossal canal
- Sphenoid bone
- Sphenoidal sinus
- Hypophyseal fossa of sella turcica
- Nasal bone
- Ethmoid bone
- Vomer bone
- Maxillary bone
- Palatine bone
- Mandible

IDENTIFY AND LOCATE

Bones in the Face

__ Inferior nasal conchae

__ Nasal conchae
                  <Superior
                  <Middle
                  <Inferior

__ Nasal comples

__ Maxilla
__ Vomer bone
__ Nasal bone
__ Zygomatic bones
__ Paranasal sinuses

LOCATE

__ Frontal, sphenoid, ethmoid, and maxillary bones each contain air-filled chambers collectively termed the paranasal sinuses.

IDENTIFY AND LOCATE

__ Frontal bone forms roof of orbit
__ Maxilla form most of the orbital floor
__ Maxilla, lacrimal, and lateral mass of ethmoid bones form medial wall of orbit
__ Sphenoid bone forms posterior wall of orbit
__ Zygomatic bone forms lateral wall of orbit
__ Palatine bone forms part of inferior wall of orbit

THE MANDIBLE

From the Lateral View

IDENTIFY AND LOCATE

__ Body of mandible
__ Mental foramen
__ Mental protuberance
__ Angle of mandible
__ Mandibular notch
__ Condylar process
__ Coronoid process
__ Alveolar part
__ Mylohyoid line

From the Medial View

__ Mandibular foramen
__ Mylohyoid line
__ Alveolar process
__ Submandibular fossa

THE HYOID BONE

IDENTIFY AND LOCATE

__ Body of hyoid bone
__ Greater horn
__ Lesser horn

Axial Skeleton

Required Instruments

| Scalpel | Blade size 22 | Saw | Blade size 10 | Retractors | Handles 3,4 |

1. Before you start, use your lab textbook and review the bones of the head, the sutures between the cranial bones, the foramina, and the corresponding vessels and nerves that go out through them—the various landmarks such as fossas, processes, etc.

2. Start by dissecting the scalp and remaining skin.

3. Use the bone saw to make a circumfereatial incision along the cranium.

4. The brain may be removed for further study through multiple dissections or left in place to remain connected to the spinal cord, which will be exposed by incising through the vertebral foramina.

5. Identify the meninges covering the brain and incise the dura adhering to the endocranium.

6. By lifting the dura, the dural venous sinuses that drain to the jugular vein will be exposed.

7. As your dissection progresses posteriorly you may identify the attachments of the tentorium cerebelli and the falx cerebri.

8. The most significant aspect of this dissection is to observe the brain and identify the points of orgin of the 12 cranial nerves.

9. Identify the:

    a. olfactory

    b. optic

    c. oculomotor

    d. trochlear

    e. trigeminal

f. abducent
  g. facial
  h. vestibulocochlear
  i. glosspbaryngeal
  j. vagus
  k. spinal accessory
  l. hypoglossal cranial nerves

Incising through the dura and lifting it completely will expose the sinuses through which these nerves exit.

THE VERTEBRAL COLUMN

IDENTIFY AND LOCATE

__ Cervical region/curvature
__ Thoracic region/curvature
__ Lumbar region/curvature
__ Sacral region/curvature
__ Intervetebral disc
__ Intervetebral foramen

IDENTIFY AND LOCATE

__ Body
__ Articular process
__ Vertebral arch

IDENTIFY AND LOCATE

__ Vertebral body
__ Transverse process
__ Transverse foramen
__ Costal process
__ Vertebral foramen
__ Spinous process (often bifid)
__ Pedicle
__ Lamina
__ Vertebral arch
__ Superior articular process and facet
__ Inferior articular process and facet

The Skeletal System and Articulation

CERVICAL VERTEBRAE: ATLAS AND AXIS

IDENTIFY AND LOCATE

Atlas

__ Anterior tubercle
__ Articular facet for dens of axis
__ Posterior tubercle
__ Posterior arch
__ Vertebral foramen
__ Transverse process
__ Transverse foramen
__ Costal process
__ Superior/inferior articular processes
__ Superior/inferior articular facets
__ Spinous process
__ Lamina
__ Transverse process and transverse foramen
__ Vertebral foramen
__ Pedicle
__ Superior articular process and facet
__ Inferior articular process and facet

Axis

__ Articulation between atlas and axia
__ Vertebral body
__ Dens (odontoid process)

From Superior and Lateral View

IDENTIFY AND LOCATE

__ Vertebral body
__ Costal facets (superior and inferior)
__ Transverse process
__ Transverse costal facets
__ Vertebral foramen
__ Spinous process
__ Pedicle
__ Lamina
__ Vertebral arch
__ Superior articular process and facet
__ Inferior articular process and facet
__ Inferior vertebral notch

70   The Skeletal System and Articulation

From Superior and Lateral Views

IDENTIFY AND LOCATE

__ Vertebral body
__ Pedicle
__ Lamina
__ Spinous process
__ Transverse processes
__ Inferior articular process and facet
__ Superior articular process and facet
__ Vertebral foramen
__ Inferior vertebral notch
__ Sacral canal
__ Superior articular process
__ Median sacral crest
__ Lateral sacral crest
__ Sacral foramina
__ Sacral cornua
__ Sacral hiatus
__ Coccygeal cornua
__ Sacral tuberosity
__ Auricular surface
__ Sacral curvature
__ Coccyx
__ Base
__ Sacral body
__ Sacral promontory
__ Ala
__ Apex

THE THORACIC CAGE

IDENTIFY AND LOCATE

__ Sternum   <Manubrium
                 <Body
                 <Xiphoid process
__ Jugular notch
__ Clavicular notch (for articulation with first rib)

RIBS

IDENTIFY AND LOCATE

__ True ribs
__ False ribs
__ Floating ribs
__ Transverse articular facet
__ Costal facets (superior and inferior)
__ Articular facets of head (superior and inferior)

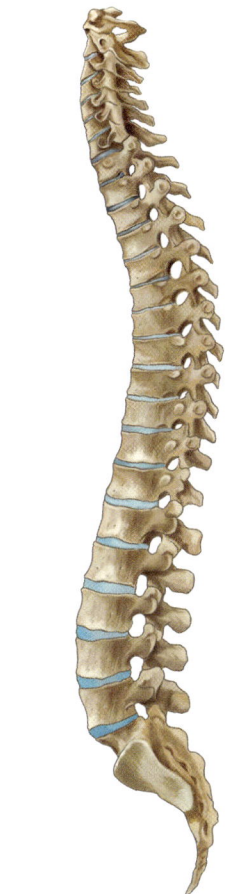

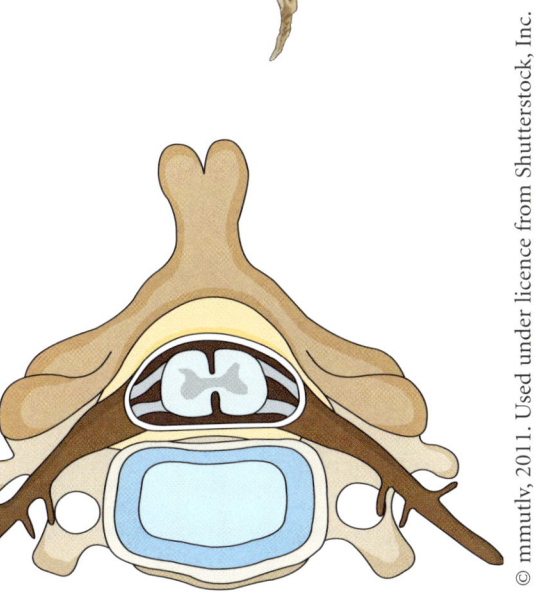

The Skeletal System and Articulation

___ Costal cartilage
___ Head of rib
___ Neck of rib
___ Tubercle of rib
___ Articular facet of tubercle
___ Angle of rib

___ Interarticular crest
___ Attachment to costal cartilage
___ Costal groove
___ Identify ribs 1-12 (from posterior and anterior views)

Name _____ Date _____

THE SKELETAL SYSTEM: AXIAL SKELETON
Laboratory Review Questions

1. The divisions of the skeletal system include which structures?

2. What bones make up the axial skeleton?

3. What is a function of the axial skeleton?

4. The orbit is formed by which bones?

5. Name the smallest bones of the skull.

6. Which bones articulate at the coronal suture?

The Skeletal System and Articulation

7. What are the bones of the facial region?

_____
_____
_____
_____

8. What are the curvatures of the vertebral column?

_____
_____
_____
_____

THE SKELETAL SYSTEM: Appendicular Skeleton

THE PECTORAL GIRDLE AND UPPER EXTREMITY

IDENTIFY AND LOCATE

__ Acromial (lateral) end
__ Sternal (medial) end
__ Sternal facet for articulation with manubrium of sternum
__ Costal tuberosity
__ Facet for articulation with acromion of scapula
__ Conoid tubercle

THE SCAPULA

IDENTIFY AND LOCATE

__ Body of scapula
__ Neck of scapula
__ Superior border
__ Superior angle
__ Medial (vertebral) border
__ Inferior angle
__ Lateral (axillary) border
__ Inferior angle
__ Lateral (axillary) border
__ Glenoid cavity

__ Supraglenoid tubercle
__ Infraglenoid tubercle
__ Acromion
__ Coracoid process
__ Suprascapular notch
__ Subscapular fossa
__ Spine
__ Supraspinous fossa
__ Infraspinous fossa

THE ARM: HUMERUS

IDENTIFY AND LOCATE

From the Anterior View

__ Head
    <Anatomical
__ Necks <Sugical
__ Greater tubercle
__ Lesser tubercle
__ Shaft
__ Intertubercular groove

__ Deltoid tuberosity
__ Lateral epicondyle
__ Capitulum
__ Trochlea
__ Coronoid fossa
__ Medial epicondyle
__ Radial foss

From the Posterior View

__ Head
__ Necks
__ Greater tubercle
__ Shaft
__ Groove for radial nerve
__ Olecranon fossa
__ Nutrient foramen
__ Trochlea

The Skeletal System and Articulation

BONES OF THE FOREARM: ULNA AND RADIUS

IDENTIFY AND LOCATE

Ulna Markings

__ Olecranon process
__ Trochlear notch
__ Coronoid process
__ Ulnar tuberosity
__ Radial notch
__ Shaft
__ Head of ulna
__ Ulnar styloid process
__ Proximal and distal radioulnar joints

IDENTIFY AND LOCATE

Radius Markings

__ Head of radius
__ Neck of radius
__ Radial tuberosity
__ Shaft of tuberosity
__ Shaft of radius
__ Attachment site for antebrachial interosseous membrane
__ Ulnar notch
__ Radial styloid process

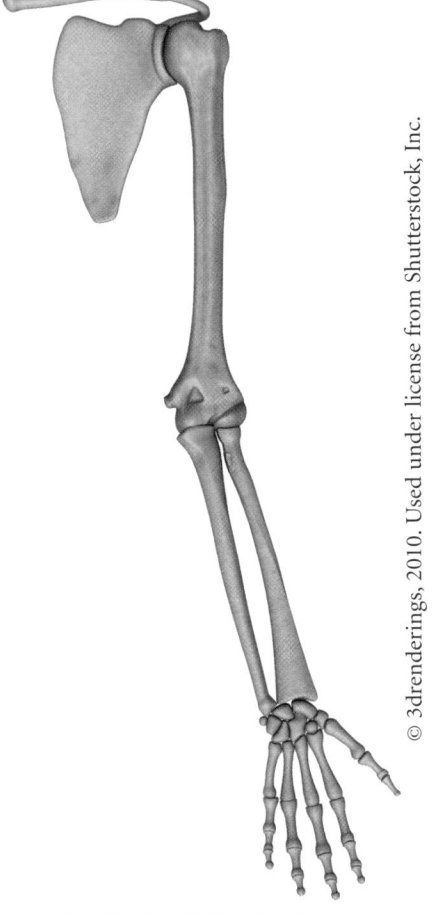

BONES OF FOREARM

BONES OF THE WRIST AND HAND

IDENTIFY AND LOCATE

__ Phalanges
__ Distal phalanx
__ Middle phalanx
__ Proximal phalanx
__ Metacarpals (I to V)
__ Scaphoid bone
__ Lunate bone
__ Triquetrum
__ Pisiform bone
__ Trapezium bone
__ Trapezoid bone
__ Capitate bone
__ Hamate bone
__ Ulnar styloid process
__ Radial styloid process

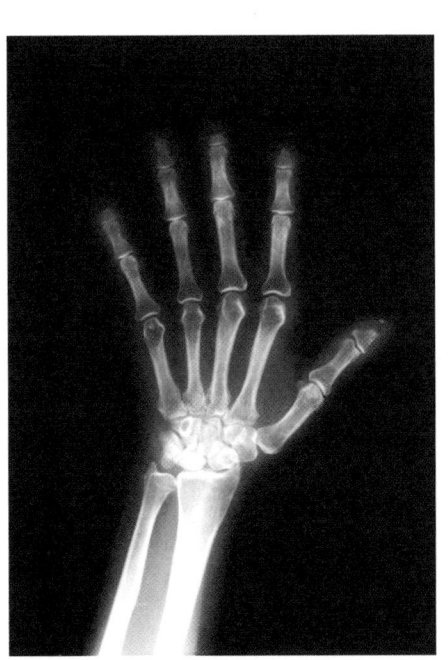

BONES OF WRIST AND HAND

Description of the Pelvic Girdle and Lower Extremity

HIP BONE: OS COXAE AND THE PELVIS

IDENTIFY AND LOCATE

- __ Ilium
- __ Pubis
- __ Ischium
- __ Iliac crest
- __ Anterior superior iliac spine
- __ Anterior inferior iliac spine
- __ Anterior gluteal line
- __ Inferior gluteal line
- __ Posterior gluteal line
- __ Posterior superior iliac spine
- __ Posterior inferior iliac spine
- __ Greater sciatic notch
- __ Ischial spine
- __ Lesser sciatic notch
- __ Ischial tuberosity
- __ Ischial ramus
- __ Obturator foramen
- __ Inferior ramus of pubis
- __ Superior ramus of pubis
- __ Pubic tubercle
- __ Pubic crest
- __ Pubic symphysis
- __ Acetabulum
- __ Acetabular fossa
- __ Lunate surface of acetabulum

IDENTIFY AND LOCATE

- __ Same structures on lateral surface visible in medial view, except acetabular structures and gluteal lines
- __ Auricular surface for articulation with sacrum
- __ Iliac fossa
- __ Iliac tuberosity
- __ Arcuate line
- __ Iliopectineal line
- __ Obturator groove

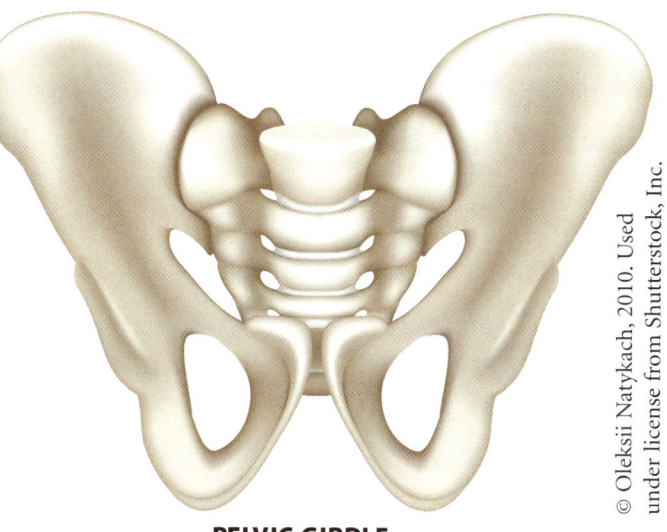

PELVIC GIRDLE

© Oleksii Natykach, 2010. Used under license from Shutterstock, Inc.

IDENTIFY AND LOCATE

- __ Pelvic inlet
- __ Pelvic outlet
- __ True pelvis
- __ False pelvis
- __ Sacroiliac (joint) articulation
- __ Hip bone (os coxae)
- __ Iliac crest
- __ Iliac fossa
- __ Obturator groove
- __ Arcuate line
- __ Iliopectineal line
- __ Pubic symphysis

The Skeletal System and Articulation

THE THIGH AND RIGHT FEMUR

IDENTIFY AND LOCATE

__ Head
__ Fovea for ligament of head
__ Neck
__ Greater trochanter
__ Lesser trochanter
__ Intertrochanteric line
__ Trochanteric fossa
__ Shaft (body)
__ Lateral condyle
__ Lateral epicondyle
__ Medial condyle
__ Medial epicondyle
__ Adductor tubercle
__ Patellar surface

Posterior View

IDENTIFY AND LOCATE

__ Same structures on anterior surface visible except intertrochaneric line and patellar surface
__ Intertrochanteric crest
__ Gluteal tuberosity
__ Pectineal line
__ Linea aspera
__ Lateral supracondylar ridge
__ Lateral condyle
__ Lateral epicondyle
__ Popliteal surface
__ Medial supracondylar ridge
__ Medial condyle
__ Medial epicondyle
__ Adductor tubercle
__ Intercondylar fossa

PATELLA

LOCATE

__ Base of patella
__ Apex of patella
__ Attachment site for quadriceps (tendon and patellar ligament-anterior surface)
                                  <Medial facet
__ Articular suface of patella   <Lateral facet

BONES OF THE LEG: TIBIA AND FIBULA

From the Anterior View

LOCATE

Tibia
__ Shaft
__ Medial condyle
__ Lateral condyle
__ Tibial tuberosity
__ Anterior margin (border)
__ Interosseous border of tibia
__ Medial malleolus
__ Inferior articular surface

Fibula
        <Head
__ Fibula <Neck
        <Shaft
__ Interosseous crest (border) of fibula
__ Lateral malleolus
__ Tibiofibular joints   <Superior
                                <Inferior

From the Posterior View

IDENTIFY AND LOCATE

__ Same structures on anterior surface visible except tibial tuberosity, anterior crest (border)
__ Intercondylar eminence
__ Medial and lateral tubercles of intercondylar eminence
__ Popliteal line
__ Articular surfaces of tibia and fibula

BONES OF THE ANKLE AND FOOT

LOCATE

__ Distal phalanx
__ Middle phalanx
__ Proximal phalanx
__ Hallux (great toe)

__ Metatarsal bones (I to V)   <Base
                                                <Shaft
                                                <Head

__ Cuboid bone

__ Cuneiform bones   <1st (medial)
                            <2nd (intermediate)
                            <3rd (lateral)

__ Navicular bone
__ Talus bone
__ Trochlea of talus
__ Calcaneus
__ Transverse arch
__ Longitudinal arch

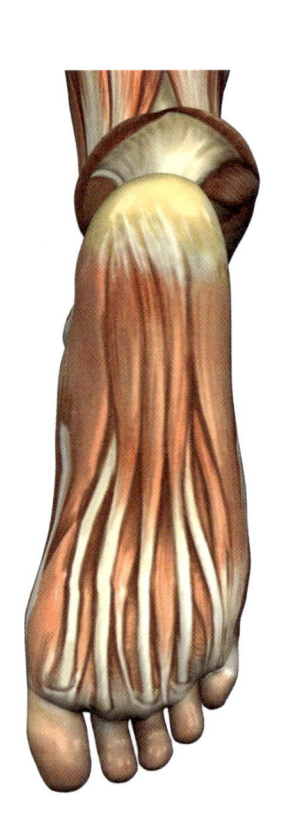

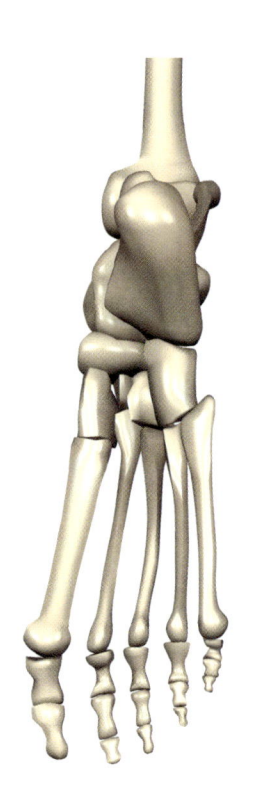

BONES OF ANKLE AND FOOT

© Linda Bucklin, 2010. Used under license from Shutterstock, Inc.

The Skeletal System and Articulation

Name _____ Date _____

THE SKELETAL SYSTEM: APPENDICULAR SKELETON

Laboratory Review Questions

1. Identify the anatomical differences between the male and female pelvis.

   _____
   _____
   _____
   _____

2. Of what does the pelvic girdle consist?

   _____
   _____
   _____
   _____

3. What is the superior margin of the hip bone?

   _____
   _____
   _____
   _____

4. What is the socket that receives the head of the femur?

   _____
   _____
   _____
   _____

5. Which bone articulates with the distal end of the femur?

   _____
   _____
   _____
   _____

6. What is the true distal end of the fibula?

   _____
   _____
   _____
   _____

7. What joints are used by a baseball player when throwing a ball?

   _____
   _____
   _____
   _____

8. Describe how a forensic scientist would conclude that a skeleton was either male or female.

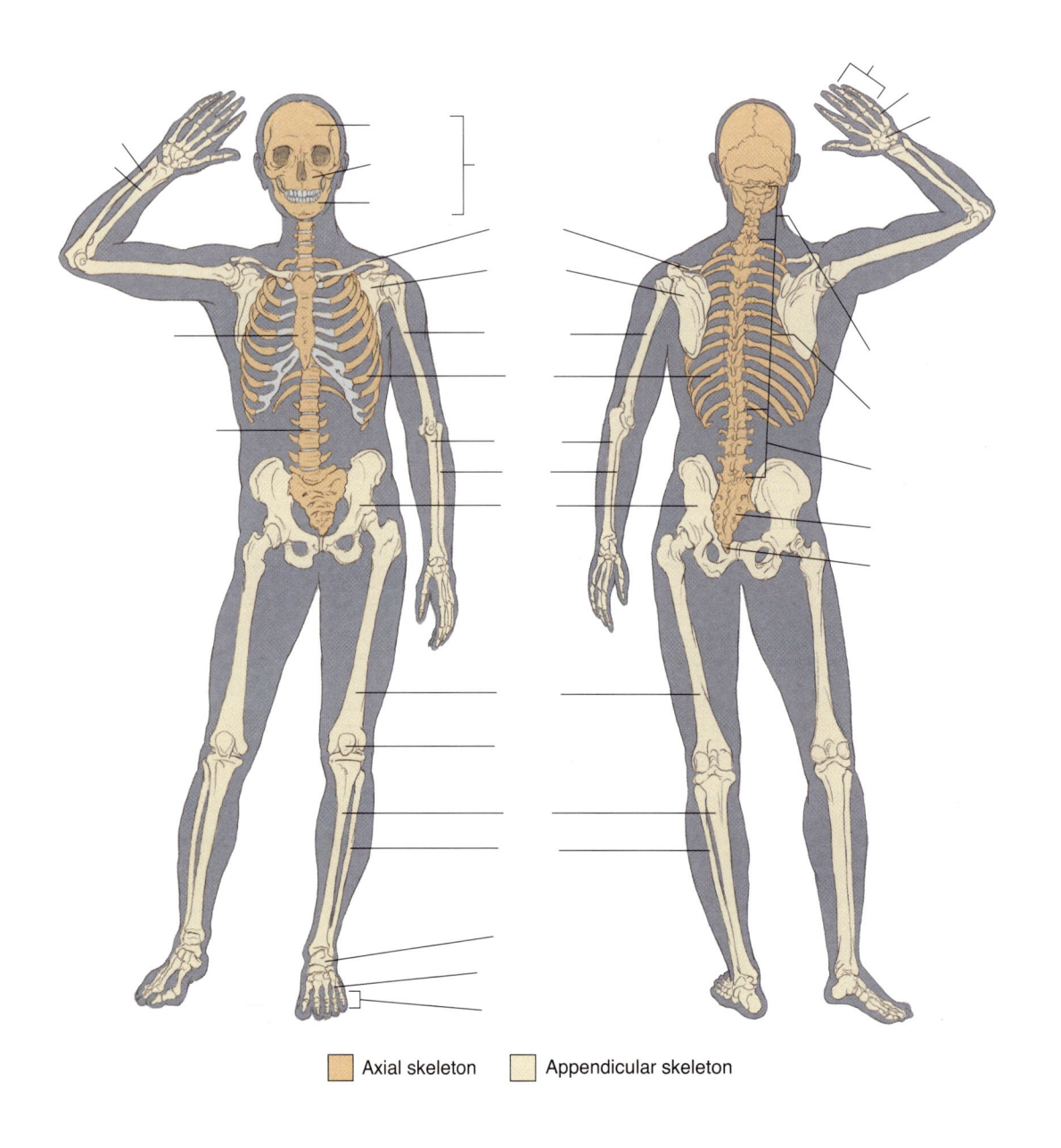

   _____
   _____
   _____
   _____

Axial skeleton   Appendicular skeleton

82   The Skeletal System and Articulation

THE SKELETAL SYSTEM: Articulations

CLASSIFICATION OF JOINTS

The junction where two bones meet is called a joint or **articulation**. The function of each joint depends on its anatomical structure. Some joints are interlocking and completely prohibit movement, others permit slight movement, while others permit extensive movement. Joints are classified depending on their structure (bony fusion, fibrous, cartilaginous, or synovial) or on the range of motion they permit. An immovable or rigid joint, termed **synarthrosis**, permits no movement because the bony surfaces are held together firmly or even interlocked (bones of the skull). A slightly movable joint, termed **amphiarthrosis**, permits a very limited range of motion (adjacent vertebrae of vertebral column). This type of joint is characterized by bands of ligaments binding bones together. An exception to this restricted movement is observed in the moveable joint between the radius and ulna.

Diarthrosis is a freely movable joint and permits a wide range of motion as in the shoulder joint. This type of joint is characterized by a **fibrous joint capsule**, a **synovial membrane** that produces **synovial fluid**, **articular cartilages** that cap the articular surfaces of the bones forming the joint, and **accessory structures**—pads of fat or cartilage called menisci or articular discs, intracapsular and extracapsular ligaments, tendons, and bursae.

INTERVERTEBRAL ARTICULATIONS

The articulations between the superior and inferior articular processes of adjacent vertebrae are gliding joints that permit small movements associated with flexion, extension, and rotation of the vertebral column. Pads of fibrocartilage, called **intervertebral discs**, separate and cushion adjacent vertebrae and form amphiarthrotic joints. The size of the disc, although variable, must conform to the size of the vertebral body. One-fourth of the length of the adult vertebral column is due to the intervertebral discs. Intervertebral discs are not found between the first two cervical vertebrae, the atlas and axis, nor within the sacrum or coccyx. Numerous ligaments are attached to the bodies and processes of all vertebrae to bind them together and stabilize the vertebral column. Neighboring vertebrae are connected and stabilized by the following six ligaments:

1. **Anterior longitudinal ligament,** which connects the anterior surfaces of each vertebral body and disc from occipital bone to sacrum.
2. **Posterior longitudinal ligament** connects the posterior surfaces of each vertebral body and disc, from C2 to sacrum.
3. **Ligamentum flavum** interconnects the laminae of adjacent vertebrae.
4. **Interspinous ligament** connects the spinous processes of adjacent vertebrae.
5. **Supraspinous ligament** connects the ends of the spinous processes from C7 to the sacrum.
6. **Ligamentum nuchae** extends longitudinally from the external occipital protuberance of the skull to C7.

Dissection Procedure

PREPARATION

Before you begin to identify the articulations between adjacent vertebrae, review the articulation between lumbar vertebrae on the articulated skeleton you may bring in to the dissection lab.

Identify the articulations between adjacent vertebrae first by observing a *model* or *skeleton* and then a *cadaver specimen*. Start your observation first by reviewing the **structures** of a **typical cervical, thoracic,** or **lumbar vertebra.**

Begin your examination of the cadaver back in the lower thoracic and lumbar regions of the vertebral column, and then move cranially to the cervical region.

Reflect the *erector spinae muscles* to see all six ligaments, except the anterior longitudinal ligament. This ligament can be observed in the lumbar region by first reflecting the abdominal viscera that covers the posterior abdominal wall. The vertebral column is still hidden by the inferior vena cava and descending abdominal aorta.

These vessels must be separated and the underlying fascia may need to be cleaned.

IDENTIFY AND LOCATE

__ Vertebral body
__ Intervertebral disc
__ Anterior longitudinal ligament
__ Spinous process
__ Supraspinous ligament
__ Interspinous ligament

Dissection Procedure

PREPARATION

Identify the following **joint structures** using first a *model* of the *shoulder joint* and then a *cadaver specimen*. To observe the shoulder joint in the cadaver, the deltoid and trapezius muscles must first be removed from the acromion and the lateral end of the clavicle.

The tendon of the long head of biceps brachii muscle and the head of the humerus are good landmarks to begin your examination.

View the joint first from the anterior. The large subacromial bursa lie superior to the tendon and humeral head; the subcoracoid and subscapular bursae lie inferior to the coracoid process.

Now locate the shoulder articular capsule as it attaches to the glenoid fossa and glenoid labrum proximally and to the anatomical neck of the humerus distally.

The interior of the shoulder articular capsule and joint cavity is best viewed from the posterior.

Clean from the posterior of the capsule any remaining muscle, ligaments, and fascia.

Cut through the posterior part of the capsule to expose the interior of the joint capsule. Locate first the articular surface of the head of the humerus and the glenoid labrum and use these as landmarks from which to identify the glenohumeral ligaments.

DESCRIPTION OF THE SHOULDER JOINT (GLENOHUMERAL)

The **shoulder joint,** otherwise known as the glenohumeral joint, permits the greatest range of motion of all the joints of the body. The head of the humerus articulates with the glenoid fossa of the scapula to form this ball-and-socket type of joint.

The **glenoid labrum** is a fibrocartilaginous structure that is attached to the margin of the glenoid fossa (cavity), completely encircling and deepening it. The stability of the shoulder joint is provided both by ligaments between the scapula and either the humerus or the clavicle and by the surrounding muscles and associated tendons. The major ligaments involved in stabilizing this joint are:

1. **Glenohumeral ligaments** lie in the anterior region of the articular capsule and are difficult to see well.
2. **Coracohumeral ligament** originates at the coracoid process of the scapula, inserts on the greater tubercle of the humerus, and is difficult to see.
3. **Coracoacromial ligament** lies superior to the capsule and bridges the gap between coracoid process and acromion.
4. **Acromioclavicular ligament** binds the acromion to the clavicle to restrict clavicular movement at the acromion.
5. **Coracoclavicular ligament** binds the clavicle to the coracoid process to prevent the clavicle from being pulled away from the scapula and to provide major support for the acromioclavicular joint.
6. **Transverse humeral ligament** straps down the tendon from the long head of the biceps brachii muscle into the intertubercular groove of the humerus.

Muscles and the underlying shoulder articular capsule are protected by a number of **bursae.** These are small, membranous sacs, which function to reduce friction and act as shock absorbers. They are filled with synovial fluid produced by the synovial membrane. The prominent **subcromial bursa** and the **subcoracoid bursa** prevent the acromion and the coracoid process of the scapula from coming in contact with the shoulder articular capsule.

IDENTIFY AND LOCATE

__ Coracoid process
__ Acromion
__ Head of humerus
__ Glenoid fossa
__ Clavicle
__ Acromioclavicular ligament
__ Subacromial bursa
__ Articular capsule
__ Glenohumeral ligaments
__ Coracoacromial ligaments
__ Coracoclavicular ligaments
__ Tendon of biceps brachii muscle
__ Subcoracoid bursa
__ Subscapular bursa
__ Subscapularis muscle
__ Deltoid muscle
__ Pectoralis major muscle

The Skeletal System and Articulation

THE ELBOW

Dissection Procedure

IDENTIFY AND LOCATE

- __ Humerus
- __ Ulna/radius
- __ Articular capsule
- __ Articular cartilage of olecranon
- __ Articular cartilage of capitulum
- __ Annular ligament
- __ Biceps brachii tendon
- __ Triceps muscle and tendon
- __ Interosseous membrane
- __ Ulnar collateral ligament
- __ Radial collateral ligament

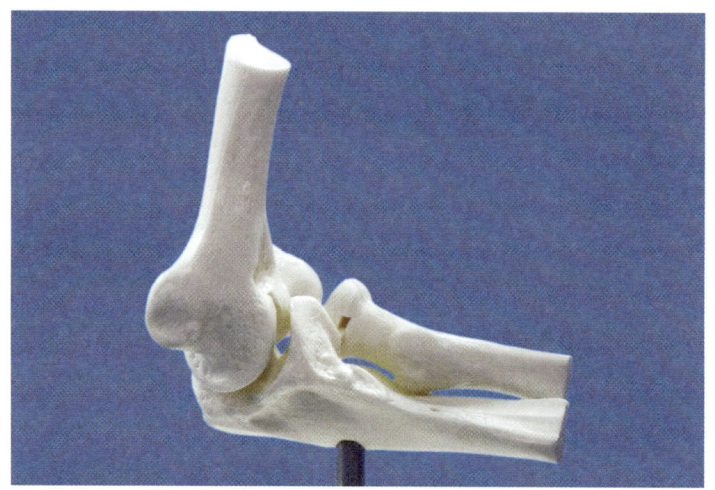

MODEL OF ELBOW

DESCRIPTION OF JOINTS OF THE WRIST AND HAND

IDENTIFY AND LOCATE

- __ Tendons from muscles of forearm
- __ Tendon sheath of flexor policis longus (radial bursa)
- __ Tendon sheath of flexor carpi radialis
- __ Common sheath of digital flexor tendons (ulna, bursa)
- __ Radial collateral ligament
- __ Palmar radiocarpal ligament
- __ Ulnar collateral ligament
- __ Carpometacarpal joint of little finger
- __ Intercarpal ligaments
- __ Carpometacarpal ligaments
- __ Interosseous metacarpal
- __ Distal radioulnar joint
- __ Digitocarpal ligaments
- __ Interosseous metacarpal ligaments
- __ Distal radioulnar joint
- __ Digitocarpal ligaments
- __ Interosseous metacarpal ligaments
- __ Midcarpal joint
- __ Carpometacarpal joint of thumb
- __ Carpal tunnel

OBSERVATION OF THE HIP JOINT

IDENTIFY AND LOCATE

__ Acetabulum
__ Lunate surface
__ Articular capsule
__ Fovea for ligament of the femoral head
__ Acetabular notch
__ Transverse acetabular ligament
__ Greater trochanter
__ Iliofemoral ligament
__ Ischiofemoral ligament
__ Pubofemoral ligament
__ Ischial tuberosity
__ Femur

__ Acetabular labrum
__ Acetabular fossa

DESCRIPTION OF THE KNEE JOINT

IDENTIFY AND LOCATE

From the Posterior View, Knee Extended

__ Femur
__ Condyles   <Medial <Lateral
__ Posterior cruciate ligament
__ Tibia
__ Fibula
__ Lateral meniscus
__ Fibular collateral ligament

IDENTIFY AND LOCATE

From the Anterior View, Knee Flexed

__ Femur
__ Fibula
__ Tibia
__ Articular cartilage
__ Patellar surface
__ Medial condyles
__ Fibular collateral ligament
__ Medial meniscus
__ Anterior cruciate ligament
__ Tibial collateral ligament

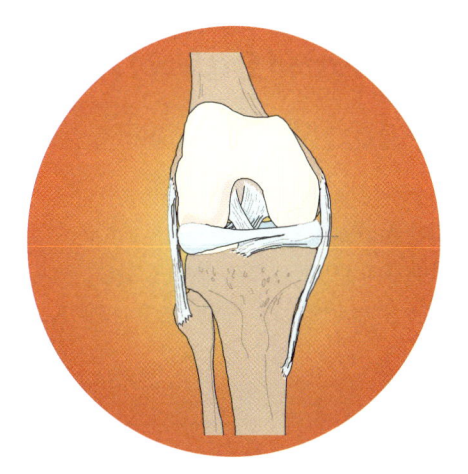

Anatomy of the Knee Joint

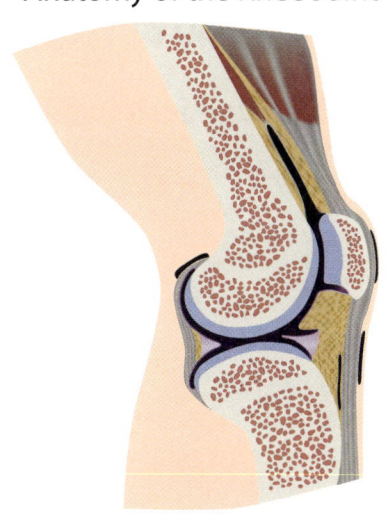

__ Lateral condyles
__ Lateral meniscus

IDENTIFY AND LOCATE

From the Lateral View

Sagittal Section

__ Femur (medial and lateral condyles)
__ Tendon of quadriceps femoris muscle
__ Suprapatellar bursa
__ Patella
__ Fat pad
__ Articular cartilage of femur/tibia/patella
__ Patellar ligament
__ Popliteal ligament
__ Lateral meniscus
__ Anterior/posterior cruciate ligaments
__ Tibia

OBSERVATION OF THE JOINTS OF THE ANKLE AND FOOT

IDENTIFY AND LOCATE

From the Lateral and Sectional Views

__ Fibula
__ Tibia
__ Posterior tibiofibular ligament
__ Anterior tibiofibular ligament
__ Lateral malleolus

__ Posterior talafibular ligament
__ Calcaneal tendon
__ Calcaneofibular ligament
__ Calcaneus
__ Cuboid bone
__ Calcaneocuboid joint

__ Intertarsal joints
__ Tarsometatarsal joints
__ Metatarsophalangeal joints
__ Interphalangeal joints
__ Talus bone

From Posterior and Sectional Views

__ Tibia
__ Fibula
__ Medial malleolus
__ Lateral malleolus
__ Tibiotalar (talocrural) joint

__ Subtalar joint
__ Deltoid ligament
__ Talocalcaneal ligament
__ Talus
__ Calacaneus

Name _____ Date _____

THE SKELETAL SYSTEM: ARTICULATIONS

Laboratory Review Questions

1. Name the suture between the parietal bones.

2. What is the significance of the hollowness of the glenoid cavity?

3. What contributes to the "opposable" capability of the thumb?

4. What is Whiplash injury? Is it hyperextension or hyperflexion?

5. List the ligaments that give stability to the vertebral column.

6. Define Primary curves.

7. The Secondary curves are the _____ and _____ curvatures formed after birth as a consequence of lifting the head and walking.

8. The action of nodding the head (as in saying "yes") occurs at the _____-_____ joint.

9. The action of turning the head side-to-side (as in saying "no") occurs at the _____-_____ joint.

10. List the 7 characteristics of Synovial joints.

_____
_____
_____
_____
_____
_____
_____
_____

11. Why does lack of exercise or inactivity weaken bones?

_____
_____
_____
_____

12. Discuss the process of bone remodeling.

_____
_____
_____
_____

13. What is a bursa?

_____
_____
_____
_____

14. What is a joint that does not permit movement?

_____
_____
_____
_____

15. What is a joint that permits a slight amount of movement?

16. The metatarsophalangeal joints of the foot resemble which joints of the hand?

17. What is a movement away from the longitudinal axis of the body in the frontal plane?

18. List the examples of angular motion and a brief description.

19. What is most likely to be the anatomical problem of a person experiencing a "slipped disc"?

20. Which knee ligament(s) function(s) to reinforce the medial and lateral surfaces of the joint? tighten only at full extension of the joint and in this position? act to stabilize the joint?

21. What are the two Bone Formation types:

    _____   _____

22. What's the difference between intramembranous and endochondral ossification.

23. Types of bone cells

24. What is the inorganic component of bone?

25. What is the organic component of bone?

26. What are the functions of the skeletal system?

27. What is a tendon? What is a ligament?

28. What is aponeurosis?

29. What is the function of chondroblasts?

30. What is the type of cartilage associated with bone function and development?

31. What is perichondrium?

32. What contains chondrocytes located in lacunae?

33. Is cartilage vascular?

34. What is proteoglycan?

35. What tends to trap large quantities of water?

36. What is appositional growth of cartilage?

37. Example of short bone, long bone, irregular, and flat bone

38. Bone regions
    Epiphysis, diaphysis, epiphysial plate, articular surface, and epiphysial line

39. What is periosteum?

40. What is the medulary cavity?

41. Where do you find the endostium?

42. What are the primary components of bone matrix?

43. What is hydroxyapatite?

44. What are chondroblasts?

45. What are osteocytes?

46. What kind of bone contains trabeculae?

47. What is canaliculus?

48. What does a haversion system contain or consist of?

49. What type of lamalae is found in osteons?

50. What bones are formed by intramembranous ossification?

51. What are osteoprogenitor cells?

52. What are centers of ossification?

53. What are the steps of endochondral ossification in their proper sequence?

54. What are intramembranous or endochondral bone growths for?

55. How do we have appositional bone growth?

56. What is the sequence of events that produce growth at the epiphysial plate?

57. Where do long bones grow in length?

58. When do they seize to grow?

59. What elements of diet are needed for normal bone growth?

60. What is the function of vitamin D? vitamin c?

61. What is the impact of sex hormones on bone growth?

62. What are the roles of PTH and calcitonine?

63. What is remodeling?

64. Stages of fracture repair in proper sequence.

65. What is the homeostasis of calcium, and what factors are involved?

66. What is Osteomyelitis and what is Osteomalacia?

67. What the difference between Osteoporosis, Rickets and Osteogenesis imperfecta?

68. Differentiate axial from appendicular skeleton

69. What is the function of the legamentum nuchae?

70. Where do you find the mastroid process?

71. What is the difference between the three types of spinal deformities: Lordosis, kyphosis and Scoliosis

72. Where do you find the dense, or odontoid, process?

73. Where do you find the transverse processes?

74. Which vertebrae do the ribs articulate with?

75. What is herniated disk?

76. What is the intervertebral disc made of?

77. What are the types of ribs and what is Sternal agle?

78. What are the parts of the sternum?

79. What girdle attaches the upper and lower limb?

80. Where do you find the glenoid fossa?

81. How many bones compose the wrist, and what are their names?

82. Which bones form the knuckles of the hand?

83. What articulates with the acetabulum?

84. If you have fractured coxa, where is the fracture?

85. What bone do you sit on?

86. What happens if a woman has a small pelvic outlet?

87. Where do you find the trochanter?

88. Which bones form Lateral and medial malleolus?

89. Which bone articulates with the tibia and fibula?

90. What is the heel of the foot?

91. How are the big toe and the thumb similar?

92. Where do you find the sesamoid bones?

93. Where is the Jagular foramen found?

94. How does tear from the eye get to the nasal cavity?

95. What is Spina bifida?

96. What the various types of joints?

97. What is the Epiphysial plate?

98. What is the Purpose of hyluuronic acid and Synovial fluid?

99. What joint is most movable?

100. How are joints named?

101. Where do you find the medial meniscus?

102. What are the 3 arches of the foot?

103. What kind of joint is the knee joint?

104. What is Osteoarthritis?

105. Describe circumduction, Rotation, Hyperextension.

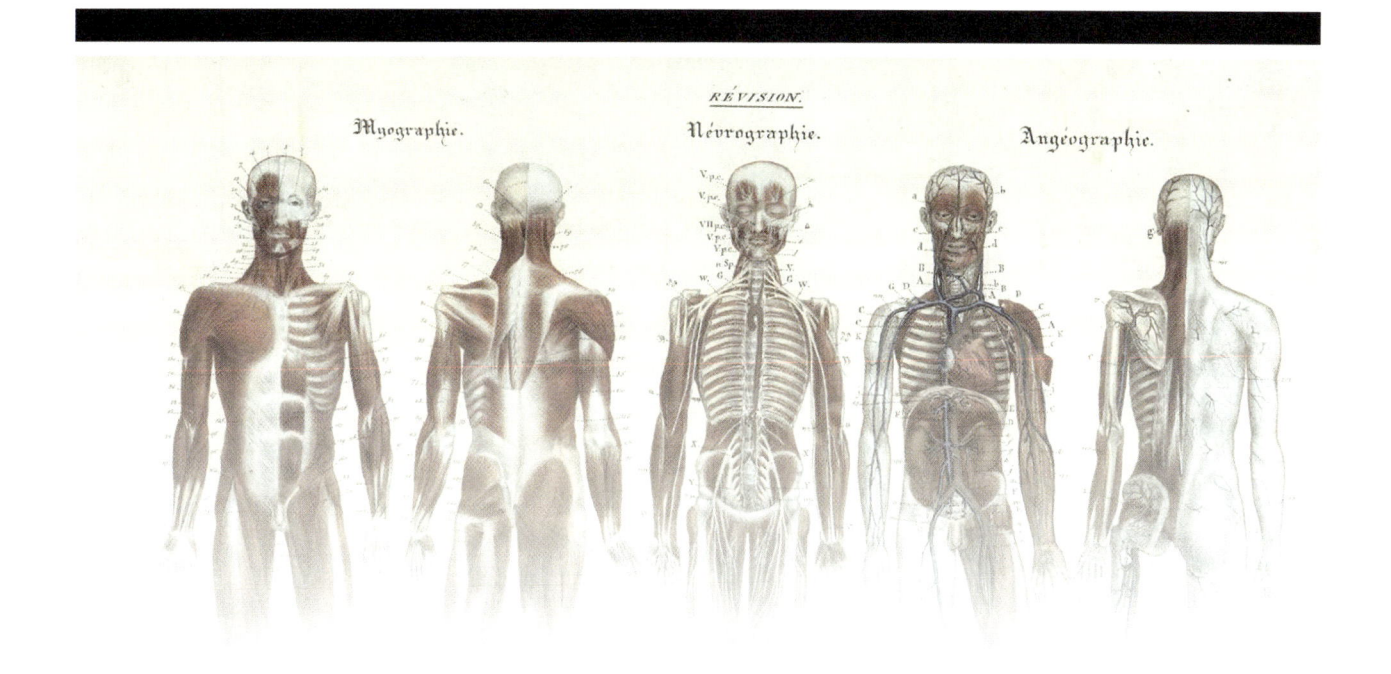

THORACIC REGION

Observation of the Thoracic Region

SURFACE ANATOMY AND PROCEDURE

PREPARATION

For the purpose of examining the surface anatomy of the thoracic region, have your cadaver lab partner stand facing you and examine the significant anatomical landmarks such as the parts of the sternum—manubrium, body, and xiphoid process, clavicle and its proximal and distal articulations—through observation and palpation. Observe the margins of the pectoralis major muscle medially and laterally. At the inferior margins of the pectoralis muscles observe the costal cartilages that form the boundaries of the thoracic cavity. Also observe your partner in a condition of inspiration along with the change the thoracic cavity undergoes during inspiration. Ask your partner to expire and observe the movements of the thoracic cavity with its muscles and various anatomical structures. If it is apparent over their clothing, observe the areolar region on male students.

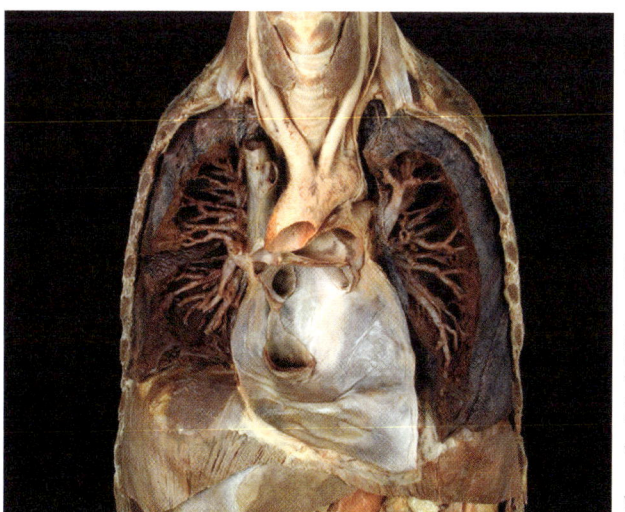

THORAX MODULE

IDENTIFY AND LOCATE

Thoracic Region (from Anterior)

__ Clavicle
__ Acromion process
__ Sternum
__ Manubrium
__ Body
__ Xiphoid process
__ Costal margin of ribs
__ Trapezius
__ Areloa and nipple
__ Pectoralis major muscle
__ Sternoclavicular joint
__ Acromioclavicular joint

Muscles of the Thoracic Region

Required Instruments

Scalpel   Blade size 22   Saw   Blade size 10   Retractors   Handles 3,4

1. Start by making a deep incision along the margin of the sternal body, deflecting the pectoralis major muscle using a blunt dissector.
2. As the pectoralis major is lifted, the pectoralis minor muscle will be distinctly identified.
3. Perform the same steps of dissection on the opposite side to expose both left and right pectoralis minor muscles.
   a. Subsequently, when you elevate the muscle fibers of the pectoralis minor with a blunt dissector, the underlying ribs will be exposed.
4. Use a sternal saw to cut the ribs vertically; this will facilitate the exposure of the thoracic cavity.
5. Along the fifth rib, the rectus sheath, which encloses the rectus abdominus muscle, also referred to as the "six pack," is exposed.
6. A similar incision should now be applied on the opposite side, which will expose both rectus abdominus muscles to the pubic symphysis.
7. On the anterolateral wall, gently incise and lift the external oblique muscle to expose the three layers of the abdominal region. The external oblique muscle's fibers extend medially and inferiorly.
8. The layer deeper to the external abdominus has fibers that run across the external oblique.
9. When the incision along the thin layer is extended, the muscle sheet can be deflected laterally.
10. Deeper to the internal oblique, the fibers of the transverse abdominis will be visible. The fibers of the muscle run transversely from the thoracic region parallel along the pubic symphysis.
11. During this dissection, the aponeurosis of these three muscles is seen to converge medially from the xiphoid process to the pubic symphysis with a characteristic white fibrous line forming the midline of the abdominal cavity.
12. This band of connective tissue can be incised to enter into the abdominal cavity and is called linea alba, which means "white line" in Latin.
13. If you are dissecting a female cadaver, make an incision around the nipple and observe where the lactiferous ducts end.
14. Continue to dissect the mass of breast tissue superior to the pectoral muscle observing the amount of fat. If the cadaver is of a younger female, connective tissue is interspaced with glandular tissue.
15. Continue the dissection to separate the pectoral muscle by making an incision along the sternal line as well as along the subclavicular margin.
16. Reflect the pectoral muscle toward the axilla.
17. Incise the skin along the axilla toward the upper arm deep into the subcutaneous layer. Initially an incision superficial to the biceps muscle can be extended down to the anticubital fossa.
18. After deflecting the pectoralis major, you will observe that the clavipectoral fascia encloses the pectoralis minor muscle.

19. Cutting this fascia along the attachment to the clavicle will expose the subclavian muscle.
20. While exposing the pectoralis minor muscle the thoracoacromial artery branches can be observed along with the lateral pectoralis nerves.
21. On the lateral thoracic wall the subscapularis insertion and the prominent edges of the serratus anterior muscle can be exposed.

The Pectoral Region

Objectives

1. Locate, identify, name, and describe the action of the muscles that position the pectoral girdle.
2. Locate, identify, name, and describe the action of the muscles of the upper limb that move: (a) the arm, (b) the forearm and hand, and (c) the fingers.
3. Locate, identify, name, and describe the action of the muscles of the lower limb that move: (a) the thigh, (b) the leg, and (c) the foot and toes.

MUSCLES THAT POSITION AND MOVE THE PECTORAL (SHOULDER) GIRDLE

Two superficial muscles, the trapezius and latissimus dorsi, cover the back. The **trapezius muscle**, which is superficial and diamond-shaped, covers the neck and most of the upper back. It originates both at the nuchal lines and in the midline from spinous processes on vertebrae C1 through T12 and inserts on the clavicle, acromion, and scapular spine. The inferior and medial edges of the trapezius muscle overlie the superior and medial edge of the **latissiumus dorsi muscle**. Expose the borders of the trapezius and latissiumus dorsi muscles. Note the location and position of these muscles and the fiber direction.

Reflect the trapezius muscle and observe the **rhomboidus major** and **rhomboidus minor muscles**, each resembling the shape of a collapsed square box. They originate on the spinous processes of the cervical and thoracic vertebrae and insert laterally and inferiorly on the vertebral border of the scapula. Deep to the reflected trapezius and superior to the rhomboideus minor lies in the **levator scapulae muscle**. Also deep to the completely reflected trapezius, the scapulae muscle overlies the superior border of the levator scapulae.

Return the cadaver to the supine position and observe the **pectoralis minor muscle**, which lies immediately deep to the *pectoralis major muscle*. The pectoralis minor originates on the ventral surfaces of ribs 3-5 and inserts on the coracoid process of the scapula. Superior to the pectoralis minor observe the **subclavius muscle**. It originates from the first rib and inserts on the inferior surface of the clavicle.

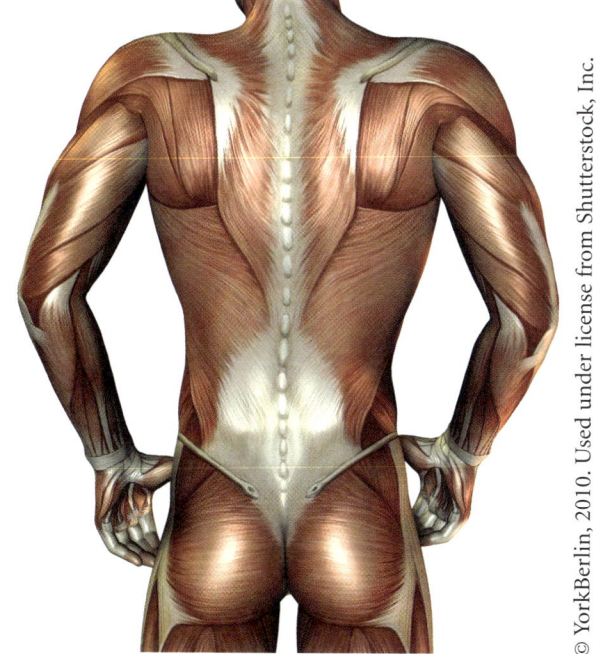

MUSCLES OF BACK

Position the arm at a right angle to the body. Reflect the pectoralis major superiorly toward the arm and view the pectoralis minor, serratus anterior, and subclavius muscles.

LOCATE

Viewed from the Posterior-
Superficial and Deep Muscles
__ Trapezius
__ Levator scapulae
__ Rhomboidus minor
__ Rhomboidus major

Viewed from the Anterior-
Deep Muscles
__ Sternocleidomastoid
__ Subclavius
__ Pectoralis minor
__ Serratus anterior

TABLE 1 *Muscles that Move the Pectoral Girdle*

Muscle	Origin	Insertion	Action	Innervation
Levator Scapulae	Transverse processes of first 4 cervical vertebrae	Vertebral border of scapula near superior angle	Elevates scapula	Dorsal scapular nerve
Pectoralis Minor	Ventral sufaces of ribs 3-5	Coracoid process of scapula	Depresses and protracts shoulder; rotates scapula so glenoid cavity moves inferiorly (downward rotation); elevates ribs if scapula is stationary	Medial pectoral nerve
Rhomboideus Major	Spinous processes of upper thoracic vertebrae	Vertebral border of scapula from spine to inferior angle of scapula	Adducts and performs downward rotation	Dorsal scapular nerve
Rhoimboideus Minor	Spinous processes of vertebrae C7-T1	Vertebral border of scapula near spine	As above	As above
Serratus Anterior	Anterior and superior margins of ribs 1-9	Anterior surface of vertebral border of scapula	Protracts shoulder, rotates scapula so glenoid cavity moves superiorly (upward rotation)	Long thoracic nerve
Subclavius	First rib	Clavicle	Depresses and protracts Clavicle and shoulder	Subclavian nerve
Trapezius	Occipital bone, ligamentum nuchae, and spinous processes of thoracic vertebrae	Clavicle and scapula (acromion and scapular spine)	Depends on active region and state of other muscles; may elevate, retract, depress, or rotate scapula upward and/or elevate clavicle; can also extend head and neck	Accessory nerve (N XI) and cervical spinal nerves

Dissection of the Mediastinum

Required Instruments
Scalpel   Blade size 22   Saw   Blade size 10   Retractors   Handles 3,4

1. Make a midline incision using a bone saw cut from the manubrium down to the xiphoid process.
2. To expand your view of the mediastinum area, incise and separate at the level of the first ribs on the right and left; next reflect the thoracic wall.
3. The heart is prominently visible at the center of the exposed space between the lungs, which is the mediastinum.
4. Continue to observe the major blood vessels.
5. The aortic arch is larger and thicker in its consistency compared to the superior vena cava where the right and left brachiocepalic trunk converge.
6. You can continue to identify the three vessels branching from the aortic arch, the braciocephalic on the left, the left common carotid in the middle, and the left subclavian on the right side.
7. Turn your attention superiorly and identify the trachea anteriorly and the esophagus posteriorly.
8. At the bifurcation of the trachea follow the right and left bronchi to the lungs.
9. The trachea compared to the esophagus has a rougher conture due the presence of the tracheal cartilaginous rings that keep it patent.
10. Continue to identify the vagus nerves and the phrenic branches on each side toward the diaphragm.

Esophagus and Posterior Mediastinum

Required Instruments
Scalpel   Blade size 22   Saw   Blade size 10   Retractors   Handles 3,4

1. After removal of the heart you may access the posterior aspect to expose the esophagus and the vagus nerves. You can identify the right and left vagus nerve branches anterior and posterior to the esophagus.
2. One of the major structures you can expose is the descending aorta.
3. With an extended incision at the diaphragm you can follow it by dissecting as it transitions into the abdominal aorta.

The Cardiovascular System

Observation of the Superficial Anatomy of the Heart

LOCATE

__ Heart
__ Right/left pleural cavities
__ Lungs
__ Diaphragm
__ Trachea
__ Esophagus
__ Bodies of thoracic vertebrae
__ Tissue of mediastinum
__ Pericardial sac
__ Fibrous attachment to diaphragm
__ Pericardial cavity
__ Pericardium <Outer layer: Parietal (fibrous)
      <Inner layer: Visceral (epicardium)

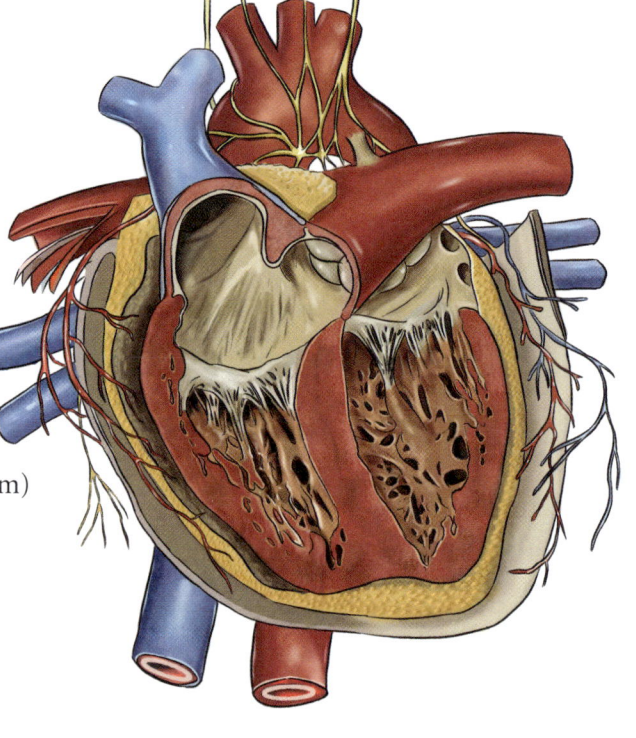

ANATOMY OF THE HEART

IDENTIFY AND LOCATE

__ Epicardium
__ Myocardium
__ Endocardium
__ Apex

__ Borders   <Superior
      <Inferior
      <Right
      <Left

__ Surfaces   <Anterior
      < (Sternocostal)
      <Diaphragmatic
      <Pulmonary

__ Right atrium
__ Right ventricle
__ Left atrium
__ Left ventricle
__ Auricle of right atrium
__ Coronary sulcus

__ Interventricular sulci   <Anterior
          <Posterior
__ Coronary vessels

__ Vena cavae   <Superior
       <Inferior
__ Pulmonary trunk

___ Pulmonary arteries   <Left
                                           <Right

___ Pulmonary veins   <Left
                                           <Right
___ Aortic arch

                                           <Ascending
___ Aorta   <Descending

___ Right atrium and auricle
___ Pectinate muscles
                                           <Superior
___ Vena cavae   <Inferior
___ Coronary sinus
___ Interatrial septum
___ Foramen ovale (not present in the adult)
___ Fossa ovalis
___ Right ventricle
___ Cusps of right AV valve (tricuspid valve)
___ Chordae tendinae
___ Papillary muscles
___ Trabeculae carneae
___ Interventricular septum
___ Pulmonary trunk
___ Pulmonary semilunar valve
___ Conus arteriosus
___ Pulmonary arteries
___ Left atrium and auricle
___ Pulmonary veins
___ Cusps of left AV valve (bicuspid valve)
___ Left ventricle
___ Aortic semilunar valve
___ Ascending aorta
___ Aortic arch
___ Descending (thoracic) aorta

LOCATE

___ Aortic arch
                                         <Right
___ Coronary arteries   <Left
___ Marginal branch of right coronary artery
___ Posterior interventricular (descending branch)
___ Anterior interventricular (descending branch)
___ Circumflex branch of left coronary artery
___ Posterior cardiac vein
                                         <Great
___ Cardiac vein   <Middle
                                         <Small
___ Anterior cardiac veins

Heart Dissection

Required Instruments

Scalpel   Blade size 22   Saw   Blade size 10   Retractors   Handles 3,4

1. After retracting the two sides of the chest cavity, expose the mediastinum and the heart.
2. Make a vertical incision at the base of the heart to detach the pericardium at the level of the diaphragm.
3. After incising the pericardium vertically deflect the flaps on both sides to expose the heart.
4. Observe the pericardial fat that surrounds the organ and provides it with protection.
5. Many cadavers will have had a number of surgical procedures done both peri- and post-mortem; observe if there are any signs of translumenal balloon angioplasty or coronary bypass grafts.
6. The size of the heart may also suggest the cause of death in the cadaver. Distention and hypertrophy of the left ventricle may be indicators of hypertension and other cardiovascular disorders during life. There may also be a pacemaker implanted or visual evidence of valvular procedures.
7. Observe the exit and entry of the major vessels.
8. The dissection of the heart could also be conducted in situ, while in the mediastinum, to observe the chambers and the valves in between them. In this manner, the tricuspid and mitral (bicuspid) valves could be clearly seen.
9. If you are dissecting the heart out of the cavity, it may be better to incise through the pulmonary trunk and the ascending aorta to fingers above their exit from the heart.
10. Insert one hand under the heart and lift it upward. In this position the right and left pulmonary vein can be incised.
11. Observe the major structures such as the right and left atrium and the corresponding ventricles. A prominent sulcus, the interventricular sulcus, can also be identified.
12. When the heart has been removed from the thoracic cavity and placed on a tray, identify the chambers, valves, and major blood vessels.

THE CARDIOVASCULAR ORGANS

IDENTIFY AND LOCATE

Artery

__ Tunica inerna (intima)
    <Endothelium
    <Internal elastic
    <membrane

__ Tunica media
    <Smooth muscle fibers
    <External elastic
    <membrane

__ Tunica externa (adventitia)

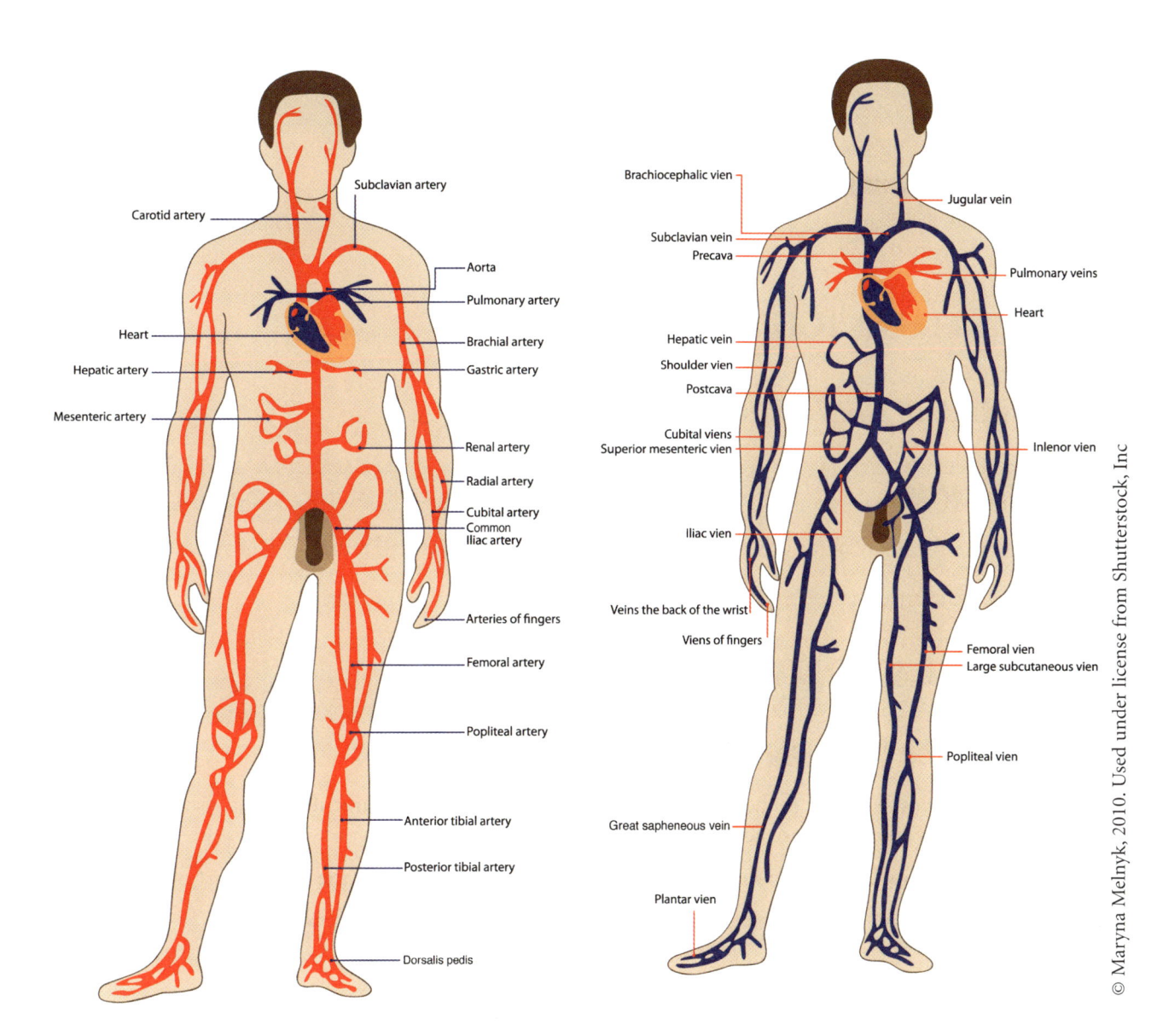

Vein

__ Tunica interna <Endothelium
  (intima)
          <Smooth muscle fibers
__ Tunica media <Elastic fibers (sparce)
__ Tunica externa (adventitia)

IDENTIFY AND LOCATE

__ Heart and chambers
__ Right/left pulmonary arteries
__ Pulmonary trunk
__ Right/left pulmonary veins

Thoracic Region

IDENTIFY AND LOCATE

The Ascending

Aorta
__ Aortic semilunar valve
__ Ascending aorta
__ Left/right coronary arteries

THE AORTIC ARCH

Observation of the Vascular System

PREPARATION

You may need to use an image or model of the circulatory system diagram in order to identify the major blood vessels.

IDENTIFICATION OF ARTERIES

Arteries of the Head and Neck

The principal arteries of supply to the head and neck are the two **common carotid arteries.** As they ascend in the neck they divide into two branches:

(1) the **external carotid,** which supplies the exterior of the head, the face, and the greater part of the neck

(2) the **internal carotid,** which supplies the parts within the cranial and orbital cavities.

The Common Carotid Artery

The **common carotid arteries** differ in length and in their mode of origin. The right common carotid artery begins at the bifurcation of the innominate artery behind the sternoclavicular joint and is confined to the neck. It arises as a branch of the right brachiocephalic artery.

The left common carotid springs from the highest part of the arch of the aorta and consists of a thoracic and a cervical portion. The **thoracic portion of the left common carotid artery** ascends from the arch of the aorta through the superior mediastinum to the level of the left sternoclavicular joint, where it is continuous with the cervical portion.

IDENTIFY AND LOCATE

__ Ascending aorta

__ Aortic arch

__ Descending thoracic aorta

<Brachiocephalic trunk
 (Innominate a.)

<Left common carotid a.
<Left subclavian a.

<Right common carotid a.
<Right subclavian a.

THE SUBCLAVIAN ARTERIES

IDENTIFY AND LOCATE

__ Major branches of the subclavian arteries
    <Thyrocervical trunk
    <Internal thoracic a.
    <Vertebral a.

__ Axillary
    <Radial a.   <Deep palmer arch
    <Brachial a.   <Superficial palmer arch – Digital a.
    <Ulnar a.

Observation of the Vascular System

PREPARATION

Since dissection of the blood vessels may be protracted in terms of the time frame for A&P at NSC, use an image or a model to identify them.

As the process of general dissection progresses, identify and locate the major blood vessels as they relate to the tissues they supply.

CAROTID ARTERIES AND BLOOD SUPPLY TO THE BRAIN

IDENTIFY AND LOCATE

__ Branches of common carotid arteries
    <External carotid a. __Vertebral   <Basilar a.
    <Internal carotid a.   arteries

__ Branches of
__ Carotid sinus
    <Posterior cerebral a.
    basilar artery<Posterior communicating a.

__ Branches of internal carotid arteries
    <Ophthalmic a.
    <Anterior cerebral a.
    <Middle cerebral a.

__ Cerebral arterial circle (circle of Willis) formed by:
    <Anterior communicating a.
    <Anterior cerebral a.
    <Posterior communicating a.
    <Posterior cerebral a.

THE DESCENDING AORTA

IDENTIFY AND LOCATE

__ Aortic arch

__ Divisions of descending aorta
- <Thoracic
- <Abdominal

__ Branches of thoracic aorta
- <Bronchial a.
- <Pericardial a.
- <Esophageal a.
- <Intercostal a.
- <Superior phrenic a.

__ Diaphragm

__ Branches of abdominal aorta
- <Unpaired Arteries
- <Celiac a.
- <Superior mesenteric a.
- <Inferior mesenteric a.

Paired arteries
Suprarenal a
Renal a.
Lumbar a.
Gonadal a.
  (Testicular or Ovarian)

__ Branches of celiac trunk
- <Left gastric a.
- <Common hepatic a_ Identify viscera and structures supplied by all the above arteries

ARTERIES OF THE PELVIS AND LOWER EXTREMITIES

IDENTIFY AND LOCATE

__ L4 vertebra
__ Terminal branches of abdominal aorta
- <Right common iliac a.
- <Left common iliac a.

__ Lumbosacral joint
__ Branches of common iliac arteries
- <External iliac a.
- <Internal iliac a.

Arteries of the Thigh and Leg

- ___ External iliac a.
- ___ Inguinal ligament
- ___ Femoral nerve
- ___ Branches of femoral artery   <Deep femoral   <Descending genicular a.
- ___ Branches of deep femoral artery   <Lateral femoral circumflex a.   <Medial femoral circumflex a.
- ___ Popliteal fossa
- ___ Popliteal a.
- ___ Branches of popliteal artery   <Posterior tibial a.   <Anterior tibial a.   <Fibular a.

Arteries of the Foot

- ___ Anterior tibial a. becomes dorsalis pedis artery
- ___ Dorsalis pedis a. branches repeatedly in the ankle and dorsal portion of foot
- ___ Branches of posterior tibila artery   <Medial plantar a.   <Lateral plantar a.
- ___ Dorsal (arcuate) arch
- ___ Plantar arch

VENOUS RETURN FROM THE CRANIUM

IDENTIFY AND LOCATE

- ___ Superficial cerebral v.
- ___ Network of dural sinuses   <Superior sagittal   <Inferior sagittal   <Left transverse   <Right transverse
- ___ Dura mater
- ___ Internal cerebral v.
- ___ Great cerebral v.
- ___ Straight sinus
- ___ Cavernous sinus
- ___ Sigmoid sinus
- ___ Internal jugular v.
- ___ Jugular foramen
- ___ Vertebral v.

SUPERFICIAL VEINS OF THE HEAD AND NECK

IDENTIFY AND LOCATE

__ Temporal v.
__ Facial v.
__ Maxillary v.
__ External jugular v.
__ Subclavian v.

VENOUS RETURN FROM THE UPPER EXTREMITIES

IDENTIFY AND LOCATE

__ Digital v.
__ Superficial palmer v.
__ Deep palmer v.
__ Palmer venous arches
__ Cephalic v.
__ Median antebrachial v.
__ Median cubital v.
__ Basilic v.
__ Radial v.
__ Ulnar v.
__ Brachial v.
__ Axillary v.

FORMATION OF THE SUPERIOR VENA CAVA

IDENTIFY AND LOCATE

__ Brachiocephalic vein (receive blood from)
    <Subclavian v.
    <Internal jugular v.
    <Vertebral v.
    <Internal thoracic v.
    <External jugular v.

__ Superior vena cava (formed by union of)
    <Left Brachiocephalic v.
    <Right Brachiocephalic v.
    <Hemiazygos v.

__ Veins emptying into the superior vena cava
    <Azygos v
    <Hemiazygos v.

__ Azygos and hemiazygos veins (receives blood from)
    <Esophageal v.
    <Pericardial v.
    <Intercostal v.
    <Mediastinal v.

THE INFERIOR VENA CAVA

Veins Draining the Lower Extremity

IDENTIFY AND LOCATE

__ Popliteal v.
           <Anterior tibial v.   <Plantar v.
           <Posterior tibial v.
           <Fibular v.   <Plantar v.

    <Great Saphenous v.   <Dorsal venous arch
__ Femoral v.   <Popliteal v.   <Small saphenous v.
    <Deep Femoral v.   <Anterior Tibial v.
                          <Posterior Tibial v.

__ External Iliac v.   <Femoral v.

Veins Draining the Pelvis

IDENTIFY AND LOCATE

                     <Right external iliac v.   <Femoral v.
                     <Right common iliac v.
__ Internal vena cava   <Right internal iliac v.
                     <Left internal iliac v.
                     <Left common iliac v.
                     <Left external iliac v.   <Femoral v.

Veins Draining the Abdomen

IDENTIFY AND LOCATE

                     <Hepatics
                                      <Left suprarenal v.
                     <Left renal v.   <Left phrenic v.
                                      <Left gonadal v.
                     <Lumbars

__ Right atrium   <Inferior vena cava
                     <Right gonadal (Ovarian or testicular v.)
                     <Right renal v.
                     <Right suprarenal v.
                     <Right phrenic v.

Observation of the Hepatic Portal System

IDENTIFY AND LOCATE

___ Inferior mesenteric v.
___ Left colic v.
___ Superior rectal v.
___ Splenic v

___ Superior mesenteric v.
___ Gastroepiploic v.
___ Gastric v.
___ Hepatic portal v.

Observation of the Circulatory System at Birth (Use textbook)

IDENTIFY AND LOCATE

___ Placenta
___ Umbilical cord   <Umbilical arteries
                      <Umbilical vein

___ Fetal liver
___ Ductus venous
___ Inferior vena cava
___ Chambers of fetal heart
___ Foramen ovale
___ Ductus arteriosus

Name _____ Date _____

THE CARDIOVASCULAR SYSTEM: VESSELS AND CIRCULATION
Laboratory Review Questions

1. What are the branches of the internal carotid artery?

2. Which artery arises from the abdominal aorta and delivers blood to the pancreas?

3. Which blood vessel type has the greatest number in the body?

4. Which vein(s) drain the cervical spinal cord and the posterior part of the skull?

5. What is a major cause of strokes that deals with a clogging of the arteries? Describe the condition.

6. What structure is present in veins that prevents backflow?

7. What is the pathway of blood into, through, and out of the hepatic portal system?

8. What is the histological makeup of a vein?

Name _____ Date _____

THE CARDIOVASCULAR SYSTEM: BLOOD

Laboratory Review Questions

1. What are the types of bone marrow and discuss their function and location.

2. What is plasma?

3. What is hematocrit?

4. Enumerate the different blood types and explain how blood-typing and crossmatching is done.

5. How does the shape of red blood cells affect gas-exchange?

6. What is the enzyme present in red blood cells that catalyzes the reaction of O2 and CO2 producing carbonic acid?

7. What is anemia?

8. How does platelets prevent blood loss?

9. Discuss the clotting mechanism.

10. What are the factors that contributes to formation of clots.

11. Differentiate thrombus from embolus.

12. What is Transfusion reaction? What causes it?

13. List the functions of neutrophils.

14. What are macrophages? what is their precursor cell?

15. What is Rh factor?

Name _____ Date _____

THE CARDIOVASCULAR ORGANS: THE HEART
Laboratory Review Questions

1. What is the cavity that surrounds the heart and contains a small amount of serous fluid?

2. What is the function of the pericardium?

3. What is the histology of heart tissue?

4. What is the pacemaker of the heart that normally sets the beat?

5. Which heart structures are involved in assisting the function of the bicuspid and tricuspid valves as the ventricles contract?

Thoracic Region 127

6. From where does the right atrium receive blood?

7. What will happen to heart function if the atrioventricular valves fail to close?

8. Draw a diagram of the heart and indicate all the internal structures you have observed during your dissection. Describe the flow of blood into and out of the heart. Include the names of the structures it passes through and where it is going.

Name _____ Date _____

THE CARDIOVASCULAR ORGANS: CARDIOLOGY
Laboratory Review Questions

1. What is preload?

2. What is afterload?

3. List 4 mechanisms how drugs may improve angina.

4. What is sinus tachycardia?

5. What is complete heart block?

6. After an infarction has occurred, certain enzymes may appear in the blood.

7. What is "end diastolic volume"?

8. What is Dicrotic notch?

9. What is Stroke volume?

10. What is the formula for cardiac output?

11. What is the effect of acetylcholine on heart rate?

12. What is the effect of NE on heart rate?

13. What is the Frank-Starling principle?

14. What would be the result of an increase in sodium and calcium permeability?

15. List 4 factors that are related to vascular resistance.

16. What is the LaPlace equation?

17. What is ejection fraction?

18. Does the AV node spontaneously depolarize?

19. What is the significance of the plateau in atrial muscle?

20. Under normal conditions, does the AV node normally depolarize?

21. What metabolic changes can one see on the EKG?

22. What do calcium channel blockers do?

23. What actually causes the first heart sound?

24. What is reflected in the 2nd heart sound?

25. In mitral and aortic stenosis, why is there a little murmur immediately?

Name _____ Date _____

THE CARDIOVASCULAR ORGANS: THE HEART

Laboratory Review Questions

1. Describe the correct order of impulse conduction in the heart.

2. Which ventricle has a much thicker wall and why?

3. Aside from the heart, what are the other structures that help facilitate venous return?

4. In the electrocardiogram, this wave represents atrial depolarization.

5. Arterial pressure is also regulated by the Renin-angiotensin-aldosterone system (RAAS). Which is physiologically active, angiotensin I or angiotensin II?

Respiratory System

Observation of the Nose, Nasal Cavity, and Pharynx

IDENTIFY AND LOCATE

__ Nose
__ Nasal conchae
__ Pharynx
__ Larynx

__ Trachea
__ Right/left bronchi
__ Lungs
__ Diaphragm

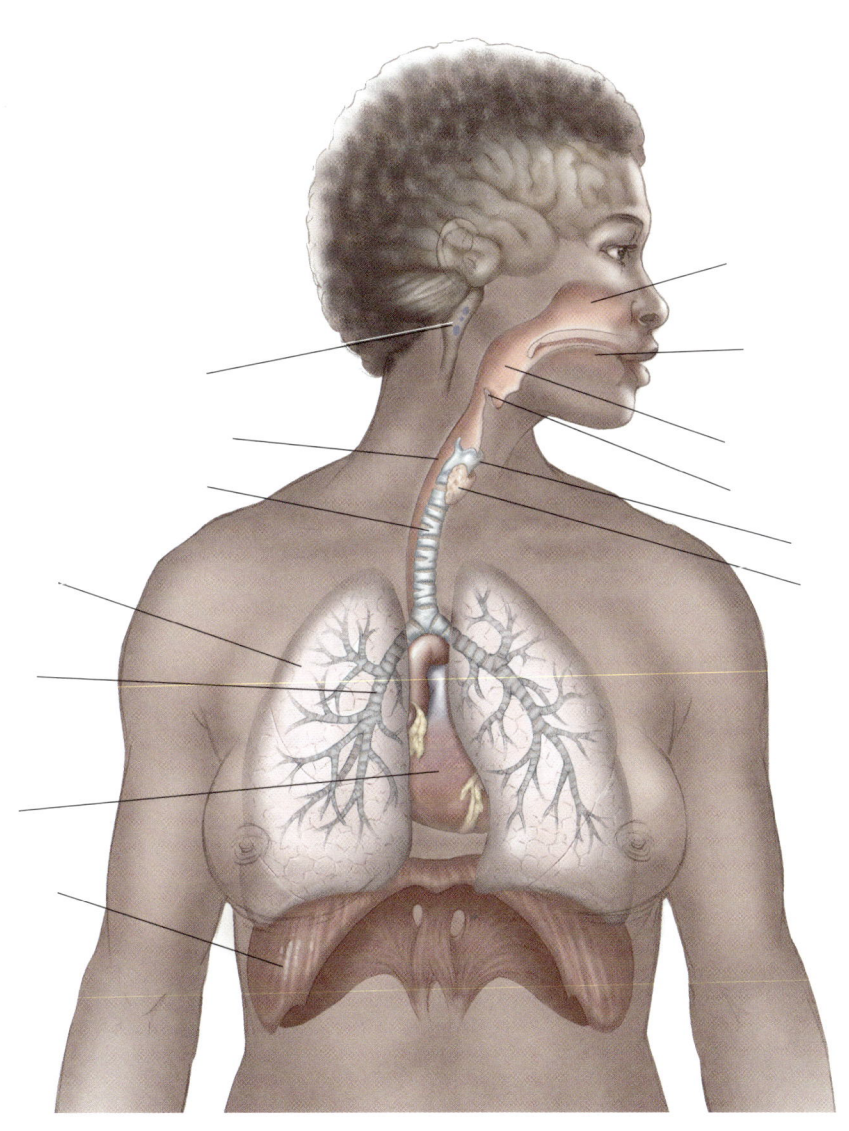

RESPIRATORY SYSTEM

Thoracic Region

Observation of the Larynx

IDENTIFY AND LOCATE

Viewed from Anterior and Sagittal
 __ Hyoid bone
 __ Larynx
 __ Thyroid cartilage
 __ Laryngeal prominence
 __ Thyrohyoid ligament
 __ Cricoid cartilage
 __ Cricothyroid ligament
 __ Trachea
 __ Epiglottis

 __ Tracheal cartilages
 __ Cricotracheal ligament
 __ Epiglottal cartilage of the epiglottis
 __ Glottis

Viewed from the Posterior
                                                <Arytenoid
 __ Cartilages   <Corniculate
                                                <Cuneiform

Observation of the Trachea and Primary Bronchi

IDENTIFY AND LOCATE

 __ Hyoid
 __ Larynx
 __ Trachea
 __ Annular ligaments
 __ Carina
 __ Right primary bronchus
                     <Superior
 __ Right lobar   <Middle
    bronchi   <Inferior
 __ Left primary bronchus
 __ Left lobar   <Superior
    bronchi   <Inferior

Observation of Superficial Anatomy of the Lungs

IDENTIFY AND LOCATE

Viewed from Anterior and Lateral
 __ Right/left lungs
 __ Apex
 __ Base
                      <Costal
 __ Surfaces   <Mediastinal
                      <Diaphragmatic
 __ Cardiac notch
                      <Superior
 __ Right lung lobes   <Middle
                      <Inferior
                      <Horizontal (Rt. Lung only)

___ Fissures   <Oblique
                        <Superior
___ Left lung lobes   <Inferior

Viewed from Medial, Right Lung

                        <Superior
___ Lobar bronchi   <Middle
                        <Inferior

___ Segmental (tertiary) bronchi
___ Hilus

                        <Arteries
___ Pulmonary   <Veins
___ Groove for esophagus

                        <Horizontal
___ Fissures   <Oblique
___ Cardiac impression
___ Diaphragmatic surface

IDENTIFY AND LOCATE

Viewed from Anterior and Lateral

___ Right/left lungs
___ Apex
___ Base

                        <Costal
___ Surfaces   <Mediastinal
                        <Diaphragmatic

___ Cardiac notch

                        <Superior
___ Right lung lobes <Middle
                        <Inferior

___ Fissures   <Horizontal (Rt. Lung only)
                        <Oblique
___ Left lung lobes   <Superior
                        <Inferior

Viewed from Medial, Right Lung

                        <Superior
___ Lobar bronchi   <Middle
                        <Inferior

___ Segmental (tertiary) bronchi
___ Hilus

                        <Arteries
___ Pulmonary   <Veins
___ Groove for esophagus

                        <Horizontal
___ Fissures   <Oblique
___ Cardiac impression
___ Diaphragmatic surface

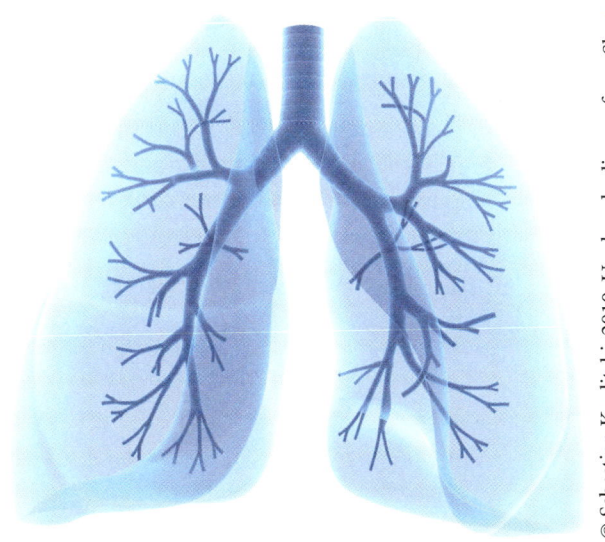

Thoracic Region

Viewed from Medial, Left Lung

__ Apex
__ Cardiac notch
__ Hilus
__ Base

                            <Arteries
__ Pulmonary   <Veins
__ Lobar bronchi   <Superior
                            <Inferior

__ Segmental (tertiary) bronchi
__ Groove for aorta
__ Base
__ Diaphragmatic surface

Dissection of the Lungs

Required Instruments
Scalpel   Blade size 22   Retractors   Handles 3,4

1. The lungs appear prominently in the thoracic cavity; observe them closely to determine the presence of dark spots, which are characteristic of smokers' lungs, tumors, or masses. These masses or tumors are distinctively identifiable when palpated.

2. Make an incision on both the right and left plura longitudinally to free the lungs and extend your hands all around the structure. You may notice some adhesion if there was an inflammatory condition.

3. During this process identify the parietal and the visceral pleura.

4. Manipulate the lungs to record their consistency by elevating them from the costodiaphragmatic recess inferiorly and laterally.

5. Based on the sheep lung dissection you have performed prior to the cadaveric dissection, identify the hilum and carefully dissect the lungs at the tracheal bifurcation and remove them from the cadaver for further dissection.

6. Identify the lobes on the right lung and the left lung.

7. The spongy consistency of the lungs reflects that it is an organ of gas exchange.

8. If you have removed the heart and the lungs to a separate tray, the thoracic cavity should appear clear to identify the descending aorta and the esophagus. The vagus nerve extends along the length of the esophagus anteriorly and posteriorly. On the right side is the azygos vein, which can be identified along with its entry point at the superior vena cava.

On the left side you can identify the ligamentum anteriosum along with the recurrent branch of the vagus nerve.

Observation of the Bronchopulmonary Segments of the Lungs

IDENTIFY AND LOCATE

__ Trachea
__ Primary bronchi
__ Lobar bronchi

Right Lung		Left Lung	
	<Apical		<Apical
__ Superior lobe	<Posterior	__ Superior lobe	<Posterior
	<Anterior		<Anterior
			<Superior lingular
			<Inferior lingular
__ Middle lobe	<Lateral		
	<Medial		<Superior
			<Anterior basal
	<Anterior basal	__ Inferior lobe	<Lateral basal
	<Lateral basal		<Medial basal
__ Inferior lobe	<Posterior basal		<Posterior basal
	<Medial basal		
	<Superior		

Observation of the Respiratory Muscles

IDENTIFY AND LOCATE

__ Scalene
    <Anterior
    <Middle
    <Posterior

__ Intercostals
    <External
    <Internal

__ Obliques
    <External
    <Internal

__ Rectus abdominis
__ Diaphragm
__ Serratus anterior
__ Sternocleidomastoid

Name _____ Date _____

THE RESPIRATORY SYSTEM
Laboratory Review Questions

1. Where are the palatine tonsils found?

2. What are the functions of the respiratory system?

3. Where is pleural fluid secreted from?

4. How many lobes are there in the right lung? The left lung? If there is a difference, explain why.

5. What are the muscles that function in respiration? Describe their function(s).

6. What is the purpose of mucus in the nasal cavity?

7. What is the opening of the larynx called?

8. Where is the actual site of gas exchange in the lungs?

9. Differentiate internal respiration from external respiration.

10. What is the product of cellular respiration? Discuss its significance.

11. Define visceral and parietal pleurae and describe their contribution in the process of respiration.

12. List the major factors that affects the affinity of O2 to hemoglobin, and discuss the significance of each.

13. What is the significance of the Bronchopulmonary segments?

14. When a person is in a sitting or standing position, where does aspirated foreign material commonly lodges?

15. A deficiency of surfactant causes the surface tension to _____, as a result, the collapsing force of the lung _____. (Choices: increase or decrease)

16. Enumerate the 3 forms how CO2 is transported in the blood to the lungs:
    1. _____
    2. _____
    3. _____

17. Differentiate Anatomic dead space from Physiologic dead space.

18. What are the 4 Pulmonary volumes and which one of these cannot be measured by spirometry?

19. How does hemoglobin (Hgb) increases the O2-carrying capacity of the blood?

Thoracic Region   143

20. How does ventilation differ from perfusion?

21. What is Aspiration pneumonia?

22. What is Pleuritis? Why is it that pleuritis of the visceral pleura is not associated with pain and that of the parietal pleura cause tremendous pain?

23. Discuss the ventilatory consequences of increased CO2 levels in the inspired air.

24. Describe the effects of physical activity or exercise to O2 exchange in the tissues and ventilation.

25. What are the immediate effects of increased altitude to respiration?

26. Define Acclimatization.

27. What is sleep apnea?

28. Compare and contrast Central chemoreceptors from peripheral chemoreceptors.

29. How will anemia affect respiratory rate?

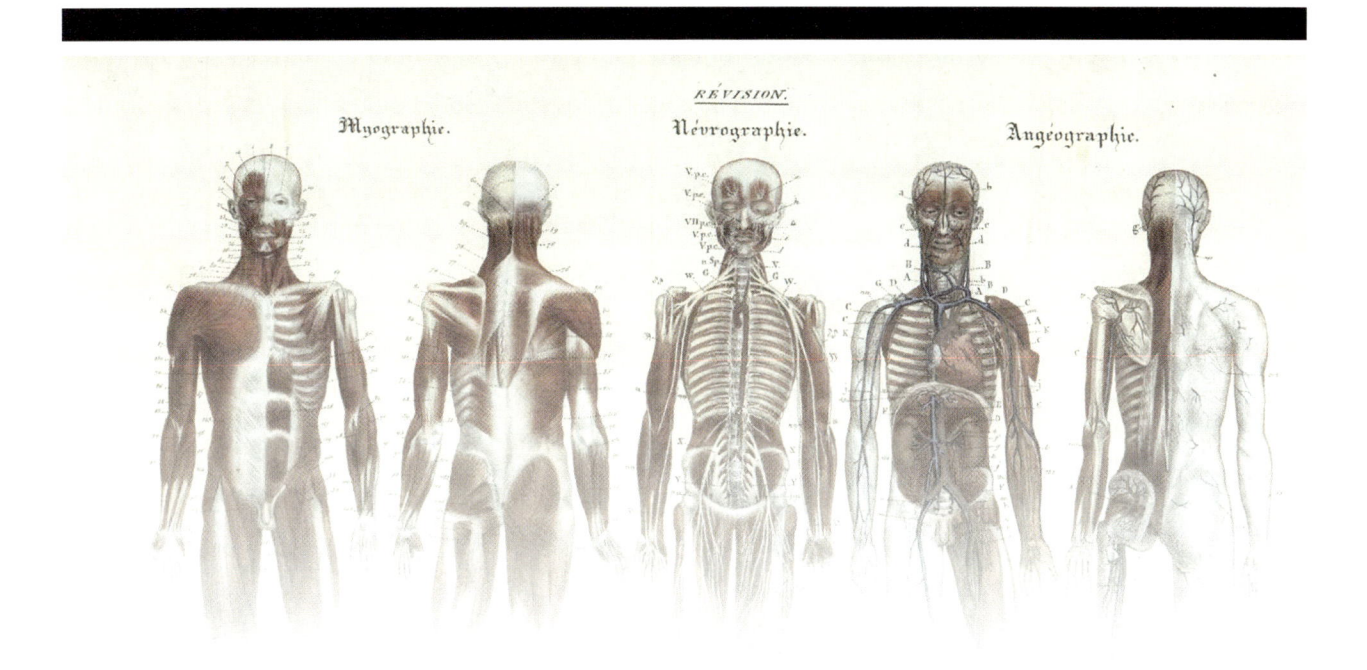

ABDOMINAL CAVITY AND DIGESTIVE ORGANS

The role of the **digestive system** in our body systems is to process the ingested food mechanically and to break down these food groups chemically using various enzymes at various levels of the gastrointestinal tract. It absorbs the nutrients contained in the food we eat and eliminates, as waste, all the undigested materials. The structures of the digestive system perform collectively the following major functions: (1) the ingestion of foods and liquids, (2) the mechanical processing of solid foods (such as the grinding of food by the teeth and mixing with the secretions of the oral cavity by the tongue), (3) the chemical breakdown of foods via the process of enzymatic digestion (such as occurs in the stomach and small intestine), (4) the absorption and processing of the nutrients released from chemical breakdown of food, and (5) the compaction and elimination of undigested and non-digestible materials.

STRUCTURES OF THE DIGESTIVE SYSTEM

The digestive system consists of a hollow muscular tube that has pouches, a coil, and bends along its length. Additionally, it has accessory organs that are connected by ducts to this tube. Accessory organs include the salivary glands, liver, gallbladder, and pancreas. The accessory organs manufacture, store, or secrete fluids that contain water, enzymes, buffers, and other components that assist in preparing organic and inorganic nutrients for absorption. The digestive system structures can be summarized as the following:

1. **Oral (buccal) cavity** contains the teeth, the tongue, and openings of ducts from salivary glands; it is the first portion of the digestive system. Grinding, moistening, and mixing of foods with secretions occur in the oral cavity. Taste, temperature, and even the texture of foods are analyzed in this region of the digestive tract.

2. **Salivary glands** secrete a lubricating and moistening fluid, termed saliva, which contains a digestive enzyme that begins the chemical breakdown of complex carbohydrates into disaccharide sugars.

3. **Pharynx** is a space that serves as a common passageway for solid food, liquids, and air. In the digestive system, it connects the oral cavity to the esophagus.

4. **Esophagus** transports food and liquids from the pharynx to the stomach. No digestion occurs in the esophagus.

5. **Stomach** performs several major functions: bulk storage of ingested food and liquids during the initial stages of digestion, the mechanical breakdown of ingested food, initiation of the chemical breakdown of food through the action of acid and enzymes, and the production of intrinsic factor.

6. **Small intestine** is the site of most of the enzymatic digestion and the absorption of water, nutrients, vitamins, and ions.

7. **Large intestine** functions primarily to remove water (dehydration), to absorb important vitamins produced by bacteria, to compact and store the indigestible and unabsorbable materials for elimination as *fecal matter*.

8. **Rectum** temporarily stores the fecal matter waste product prior to elimination.

9. **Pancreas** exocrine cells secrete buffers and digestive enzymes; endocrine cells secrete hormones.

10. **Liver** secretes bile (required for emulsification and subsequent digestion of fats), stores nutrients and vitamins, and has many metabolic and regulatory functions.

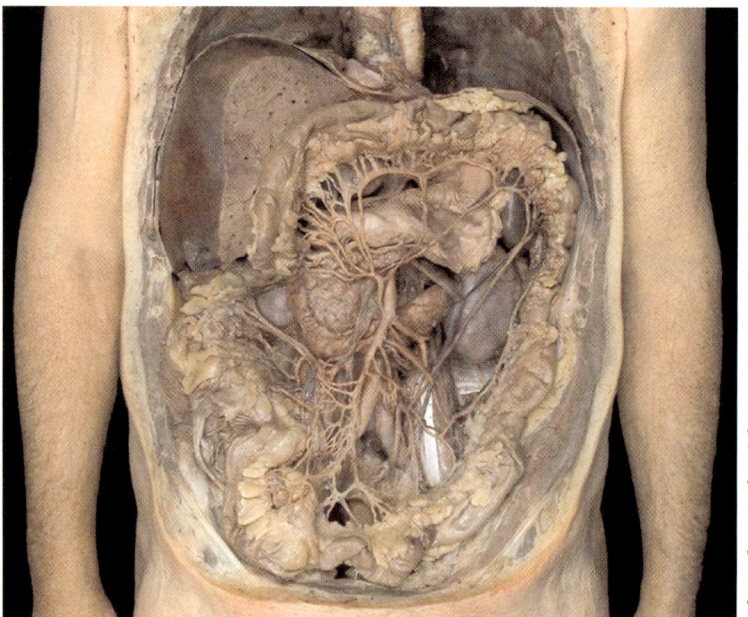

11. **Gallbladder** stores and concentrates bile that it receives from the liver. Under hormonal and nervous system control, bile drains from the gallbladder into the small intestine.

PROCEDURE

Identify the structures that compose the **digestive tract** and **accessory organs** on the torso model. Begin by removing the chest plate and the detachable head/neck section from the intact torso. Head and neck structures are now viewed in mid-sagittal section. Next remove the heart and lungs from the thoracic cavity. Identify the **oral (buccal) cavity, salivary glands, esophagus, stomach, small intestine, large intestine,** and **rectum**. Now identify the accessory organs—**liver, gallbladder,** and **pancreas**.

Review the **abdominal regions** on the torso or cadaver. It is important to have a mental picture of the shape, size, and organization of the digestive organs within their respective abdominal regions because descriptions of their location and relationships are based upon this regional terminology.

IDENTIFY AND LOCATE

__ Oral (buccal) cavity
__ Salivary glands
__ Esophagus
__ Stomach
__ Small intestine
__ Large intestine
__ Rectum
__ Liver
__ Gallbladder
__ Pancreas

Abdominal Regions
__ Right/left hypochondriac regions
__ Epigastric region
__ Right/left lumbar regions
__ Umbilical
__ Right/left iliac regions
__ Hypogastric region

Abdominal Cavity

Required Instruments
Scalpel   Blade size 22   Saw   Blade size 10   Retractors   Handles 3,4

1. Once the abdominal cavity is entered by incising the peritoneum, you will identify the fatty apron covering the abdominal viscera known as the greater omentum.

2. Deflect the greater omentum superiorly by manipulating the hepatoduodenal and hepatogastric ligaments to expose the abdominal organs.

3. The liver is located on the right hypochondial region and where you can identify the two lobes separated by the falciform ligament and the round ligament inferiorly.

4. Turn the liver superiorly by dissecting the triangular and the coronary ligaments that have attached it to the diaphragm; you can now observe the gall bladder, if present.

5. Using hemostats attempt to separate and identify the junction of the cystic duct into the common bile duct.

6. Follow the common bile duct superiorly and you will observe the hepatic branch.

7. Turn your attention to the duodenum to identify the point of contact with the pancreas.

8. You can gently dissect the gall bladder from the hepatic fossa and remove it from the cadaver for subsequent dissections on a tray.

9. Dissect the gall bladder to observe if there are gall stones. You may also observe the color and consistency of bile.

10. You may also identify the entry point of the hepatic veins at the vena cava.

11. Lift the stomach slightly and identify the greater and lesser curvatures.

12. Distally, identify the pyloric sphincter by palpation as the muscular layer is thicker than the rest of the stomach.

13. Distal to the pyloric sphincter the duodenum can be identified and at the duodeno jejunal junction the suspensory ligament (treitz) is identified.

14. Continue along the length of the intestines and identify the fan-like structure, which is the mesentery.

Spread the mesentery to observe the blood vessels and lymphatic nodules that appear as dots on this semi-transparent tissue.

15. Follow the length of the intestine to the ileocecal junction. Identify the cecum and if there was no appendectomy, the vermiform appendix can be located at the blind pouch of the cecum.

16. The cecum superiorly continues as the ascending colon and, at the level of the liver, it forms the hepatic flexure to continue as the transverse colon.

17. Observe the structure difference of the colon from the small intestine.

18. Observe the haustra, the pouch-like segement of the colon and tenie coli.

19. Continue dissecting the transverse colon as it forms a curvature at the the level of the splenic flexure.

20. Dissection can now continue along the colon to the pelvic cavity where you will identify the sigmoid colon and the rectum.

21. To avoid spilling the contents of the colon and the stomach, it may be a better option to ligate the stomach at the cardiac/gastroesopageal sphincter and dissecting, and concurrently figating and dissecting the rectum at the level of the anus.

22. Remove the entire content of the GI tract and place it on a tray for further dissection if the cadaver is preserved in an immersive container.

23. Continue dissection on a tray and expose the inner lining of the stomach and rugae.

24. Expose the inner surface of the duodenum to observe the choledochoduodenal sphincter and the pancreatic duodenal sphinter/sphincter of Oddi.

LAYERS OF THE DIGESTIVE TRACT

The digestive tract is organized as a four-layered tube. These layers are continuous along the entire length of the tube but are modified within specified organs reflecting the special digestive activities that occur in these organs. These structural modifications determine the function of each of these digestive organs. Modifications create a division of labor among the digestive organs, with each organ playing a specific role in the overall digestive process. The four layers (tunics) of the digestive tube are best identified from inside to out.

Mucosa is the innermost layer that lines the lumen of the digestive tube. This layer is composed of an epithelium moistened by glandular secretions and sometimes organized into pleats and folds. Folds increase surface area for digestion and absorption. They also permit expansion of the diameter of the digestive tube to accommodate foods for their passage through the tube lumen. The mucosa of the oral cavity and esophagus has a stratified squamous epithelium. It changes to columnar epithelium in the stomach and small and large intestines, and then back to stratified squamous epithelium in the last part of the rectum. An underlying lamina propria always forms the connective tissue basement foundation for the mucosa. A narrow band of smooth muscle fibers, muscularis mucosae, is located in most areas of the digestive tract along the outer portion of the lamina propria.

Submucosa is the layer that contains dense connective tissue that serves to support the blood vessels, nerves, and lymphatics that service each structure of the digestive tube. In some regions, the submucosa has exocrine glands that secrete products into the lumen of the digestive tract to aid in digestion (e.g., mucous glands, esophagus).

Muscularis externa is the layer that contains smooth muscle fibers organized into longitudinal and circular bands for the movement of foodstuffs through the digestive tube. The longitudinal band forms the outer muscle layer and runs the length of the tube. When contracted, a portion of the tube shortens. The circular band wraps around the tube and forms the inner muscle layer. Contracting this band causes the diameter of the tube to be constricted. In the stomach only, an oblique band is the innermost smooth muscle layer.

Under the control of the ANS, the contraction of these smooth mucle bands promotes the movement of chyme through the digestive tube and compartmentalizes it. It is the arrangement of smooth muscle layers, the contractile properties of smooth muscle cells, and control by the ANS that produces slow, sustained contractions known as **peristalsis**. Peristalsis occurs because of the coordinated contractions of longitudinal and circular muscle layers, which results in the slow movement of contents through the lumen of the digestive tract. A more specialized movement, termed **segmentation**, occurs within the small and large intestines to mix foods with digestive secretions. Segmentation movements predominantly involve the circular muscle layer, serving not only to mix chime but also to fragment and compact it.

Serosa is the layer that is the visceral peritoneum. The peritoneum is a serous membrane consisting of two portions: a visceral layer that covers each abdominal organ and a parietal layer that lines the abdominal cavity. The peritoneal fluid formed on the surfaces of these membranes prevents friction between the body walls and organ surfaces. A connective tissue layer of collagen fibers, termed the **adventitia**, attaches the oral cavity, esophagus, and rectum to surrounding structures.

IDENTIFY AND LOCATE

__ Mucusoa
       <Mucous epithelium
       <Lamina propria
       <Muscularis mucosae

__ Muscularis externa
       <Circular muscular layer (inner)
       <Longitudinal muscle layer (outer)

__ Plica (mucosal fold)
__ Submucosa

__ Serosa

Observations of the Serous (Peritoneal) Membranes

Segments of the digestive tract are suspended within the peritoneal cavity by the visceral peritoneum (serosa) covering these segments. Laminating the visceral and parietal peritoneal membranes together creates the **serous membranes**. Serous membranes are named according to the location and organs suspended. For example, the serous membrane connected with the large intestine is termed mesocolon. The serous membrane of the small intestine, termed **mesentery**, serves to attach it to the posterior body wall and to connect its coils together thereby preventing strangulation by the twisting of blood vessels, lymphatics, and nerves that supply the small intestine.

DISSECTION PROCEDURE

1. The **serous membranes** that support the digestive tract and attack the visceral organs to the posterior peritoneal wall using a torso model or cadaver specimen. Note, a torso model will not depict all of the serous membranes; only a cadaver specimen contains all serous membranes.

2. Identify the serosa lining of the abdominal wall as the parietal peritoneum. Observe the fold of serous membrane between the liver and the stomach as the **lesser omentum**. (Typically not present on models.)

3. Locate the greater curvature of the stomach and identify the **greater omentum** as the curtain of serous membrane with fat that drapes over the intestines. (Only a portion depicted on models.) The greater omentum is a large fold of the dorsal mesentery of the stomach that drapes and hangs anterior to the intestines. "Pot bellies" are the result of the accumulation of large amounts of fat within the greater omentum. Recall that the abdominal wall is formed only by skin and four layers of muscle. It does not contain any bony areas for protection (except for L1-5 vertebrae and pelvis). Both omenta serve to protect the abdominal organs and provide a storage area for fat until it is required for metabolism.

4. Locate the diaphragm and liver. Identify the **falciform ligament** as the serous membrane that suspends the liver from the anterior abdominal wall and inferior surface of the diaphragm. It appears as a white

line on the anterior surface of the liver, dividing it into right and left lobes. Trace the ligament superiorly and note that it splits.

5. Identify the right division as the **coronary ligament** of the liver (appears as a white line of all models). In life, the coronary ligament encases the right lobe of the liver. Locate the small intestine and identify the **mesentery proper**, which suspends the small intestine from the posterior body wall via the **root of the mesentery proper**.

6. Locate the large intestine and identify that portion that passes in a transverse place as the transverse mesocolon. The **mesocolon** suspends this portion of the large intestine at its dorsal surface to the posterior body wall. The remaining portions are also suspended by mesocolon and are described with the large intestine.

LOCATE

__ Parietal peritoneum
__ Mesentery (proper) of the small intestine
__ Lesser omentum
__ Greater omentum
__ Root of the mesentery proper
__ Falciform ligament
__ Coronary ligament of liver
__ Mesocolon

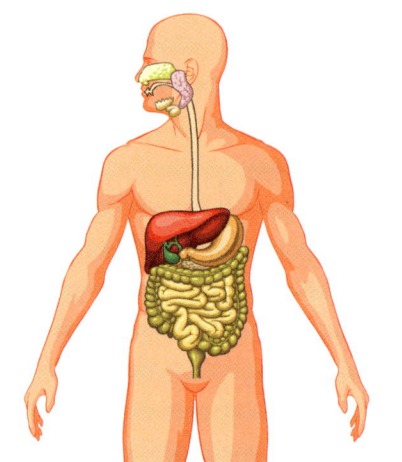

Observation of Oral (Buccal) Cavity Structures and Pharynx

As described earlier, the oral (buccal) cavity contains the teeth, openings of ducts to the salivary glands, and tongue. It is the first part of the digestive system and is lined by the **oral mucosa**, which is a stratified squamous epithelium. The oral cavity is continuous with the *pharynx*, which is the common passageway for foods, liquids, and air.

DISSECTION PROCEDURE

Since this procedure may be difficult to perform on the cadaver itself, identify the following structures of the **oral (buccal) cavity** using your lab partner's body, torso model, and cadaver specimen. View through the open mouth the structures of the oral cavity on your partner or use a mirror to observe them on yourself. Identify the teeth, floor, and roof of the oral cavity. The floor contains the tongue and the openings of the ducts of most of the salivary glands. Differentiate between the **hard** and **soft palates** by running the tip of your tongue over the roof of the oral cavity. The palatine process of the maxillary bone and the palatine bone form the hard palate. The soft palate begins immediately posterior to the palatine bone and can be felt as the "soft" portion of the roof. Identify a pendulous extension in the midline, the **uvula**, at the posterior of the soft palate. Identify the **palatopharyndeal arches** as muscular arches of the soft palate, which frame the oral cavity and form a boundary between it and the oropharynx. Posterior to the arches a pair of palatine tonsils can be identified. These tonsils are typically visible. If not, they may have been surgically removed.

The majority of the space in the oral cavity is occupied by the **tongue**. Recall that the muscular tongue is covered by stratified squamous epithelium. Observe the superior surface of the tongue, the **dorsum**, and note the numerous papillae that appear only on this surface. Identify the portion of the tongue anterior to the palatoglossal arch as the **body**, and the portion located posterior to the arch as the **root**. In the midline, on the inferior surface of the tongue, identify a fold of mucous membrane, the **lingual frenulum**, which secures the tongue to the floor of the oral cavity. Identify on the floor lateral to the frenulum the openings of submandibular ducts. These ducts transport saliva from the submandibular glands to the floor of the oral cavity.

IDENTIFY AND LOCATE
Viewed through the Open Mouth

__ Teeth
__ Hard/Soft palates
__ Uvula
__ Palatoglossal arches
__ Palatine tonsils

__ Tongue   <Dorsum
                <Body
                <Root

__ Papillae
__ Lingual frenulum
__ Openings of submandibular ducts

Viewed in Sagittal Section

__ All of the mentioned structures
__ Cheek (oral mucosa) may be seen in section, except submandibular ducts
__ Nasal/oral cavities

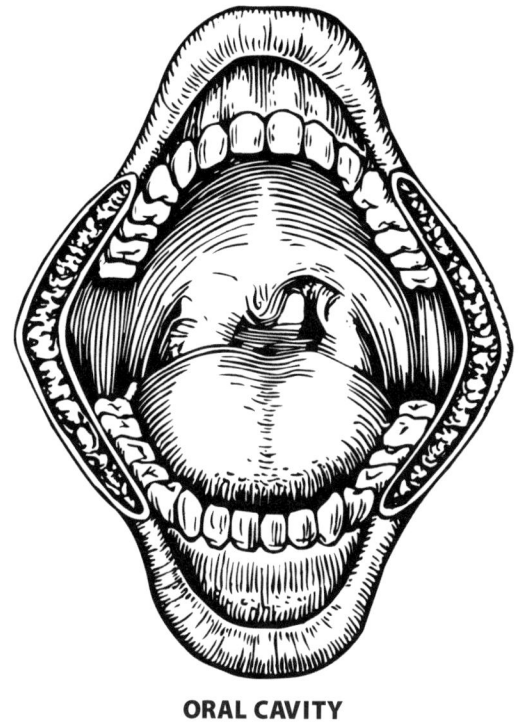

__ Pharynx   <Nasopharynx
                  <Oropharynx
                  <Laryngopharynx

ORAL CAVITY

__ Lips
__ Vestibule
__ Gingiva (gums)

__ Opening to parotid duct
__ Entrance to auditory tube

Observation of the Salivary Glands

IDENTIFY AND LOCATE

__ Parotid gland
__ Parotid duct
__ Submandibular glands
__ Submandibular ducts
__ Sublingual gland
__ Sublingual ducts

IDENTIFY AND LOCATE

__ Serous cells
__ Mucous cells
__ Ducts
__ Blood vessels

LOCATE

__ Incisors (medial/lateral)
__ Cuspids (canines)
__ Bicuspids (premolars)
__ Molars
__ Crown
__ Root
__ Neck
__ Enamel
__ Dentin
__ Pulp cavity
__ Gingiva
__ Gingival sulcus
__ Peridontal ligament (membrane)
__ Bone of alveolus
__ Root canal
__ Apical foramen
__ Branches of alveolar vessels and nerve

IDENTIFY AND LOCATE

__ Laryngopharynx
__ Trachea
__ Esophagus
__ Diaphragm

__ Esophageal hiatus
__ Stomach
__ Vagus nerves

__ Blood vessels   <Esophageal a./v.
                  <Azygos v.

IDENTIFY AND LOCATE

External Anatomy

__ Relation of
    <Diaphragm
    <Esophagus
    <Liver

__ Greater omentum

<Fundus

__ Surface of stomach
    <Anterior, posterior,
    <medial, and lateral
    <Greater curvature
    <Lesser curvature

__ Stomach regions
    <Cardia
    <Body
    <Pylorus

__ Lesser omentum
    <Hepatoduodenal
    <Ligament
    <Hepatogastric
    <ligament

__ Celiac Artery
    <Left gastric a.
    <Common hepatic a.
    <Splenic a.

Internal Anatomy

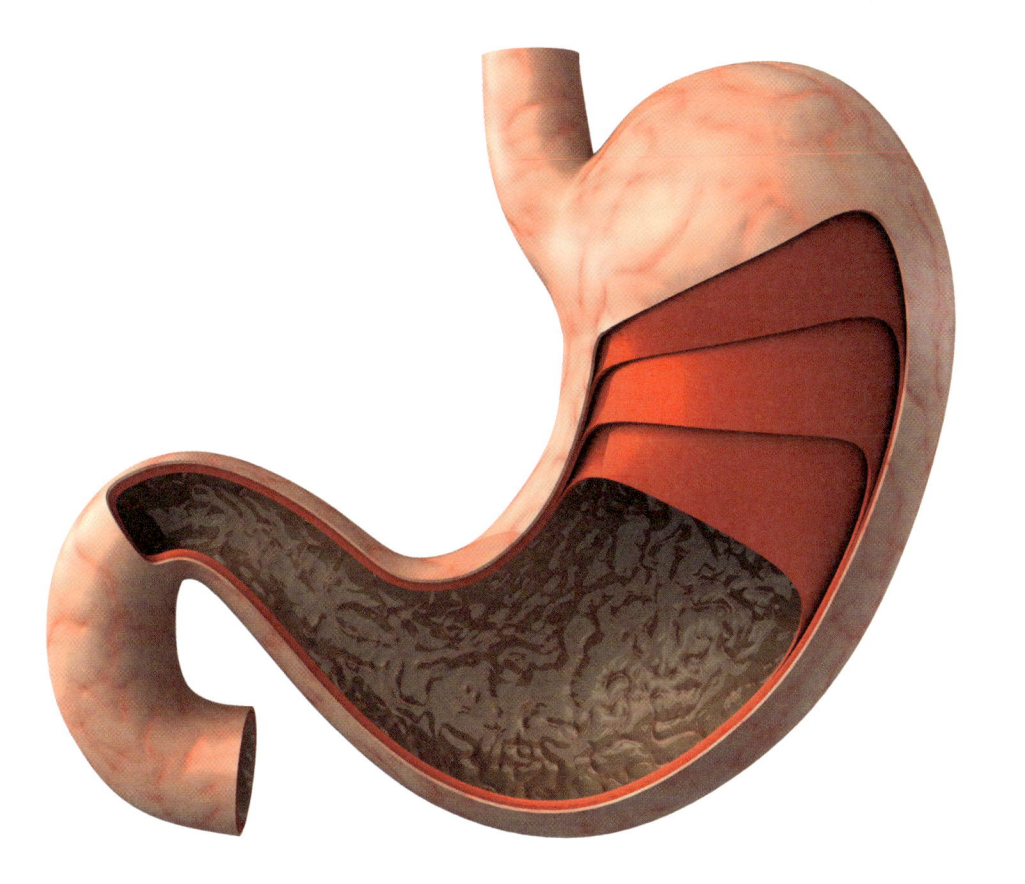

__ Stomach regions
__ Cardiac orifice and esophageal lumen
__ Pyloric sphincter
__ Pyloric orifice

__ Rugae

__ Muscular layers   <Longitudinal (outer)
                      <Circular (middle)
                      <Oblique (inner)

ANATOMY OF STOMACH

GROSS ANATOMY OF THE SMALL INTESTINE

IDENTIFY AND LOCATE

__ Position of small intestine abdominopelvic cavity and relation to other abdominal organs
__ Pyloric sphincter of stomach
__ Duodenum
__ Jejunum
__ Ileum
__ Ileocecal valve

Mesentery
__ Mesentery proper
__ Root of mesentery

Blood Vessels
__ Abdominal aorta
__ Superior mesenteric artery/vein contained in mesentery proper
__ Hepatic portal vein

Observation of the Large Intestine

IDENTIFY AND LOCATE

__ Large intestine
__ Epiploic appendage flexure
__ Haustra
__ Taenia coli
__ Ileocecal valve
__ Cecum
__ Appendix
__ Ascending colon
__ Right colic (hepatic) flexure

__ Transverse colon
__ Left colic (splenic)
__ Anal
__ Descending colon orifice
__ Sigmoid colon
__ Rectum
__ Anal canal
__ Anal columns
__ Internal/external anal sphincters

__ Anus

Blood Supply
__ Superior mesenteric artery/vein
__ Inferior mesenteric artery/vein

Observation of the Liver and Gallbladder

IDENTIFY AND LOCATE

Viewed from the Anterior

(Parietal) Surface

__ Right/left liver lobes
__ Falciform ligament
__ Coronary ligament
__ Round ligament (ligamentum teres)

Viewed from the Posterior (Visceral) Surface

__ Falciform ligament
                              <Caudate lobe
__ Right liver lobe   <Quadratic lobe
__ Left liver lobe
__ Porta hepatis
__ Inferior vena cava
__ Hepatic artery proper
__ Branches of hepatic portal vein

Gallbladder

__ Regions of gallbladder   <Fundus
                              <Body
                              <Neck

__ Cystic duct
__ Spiral valve (of Heister—not readily visible)
__ Left/right hepatic ducts
__ Common bile duct

__ Duodenal   <Common bile duct
   papilla   <Pancreatic duct
   within   <Duodenal (major)
   duodenum   < ampulla
                       <Hepatopancreatic
                       < sphincter

IDENTIFY AND LOCATE

                       <Head   __ Accessory duct (duct of Santorini)
__ Regions of pancreas   <Body   __ Hepatopancreatic sphincter (of Oddi)
                       <Tail
__ Pancreatic duct (duct of Wirsung)

IDENTIFY AND LOCATE

__ Stomach   __ Pancreaticoduodenal artery
                     <Head   __ Pancreatic artery
__ Pancreas   <Body   __ Celiac trunk artery
                     <Tail   __ Superior mesenteric artery

__ Duodenum
__ Abdominal aorta
__ Celiac trunk

Abdominal Cavity and Digestive Organs

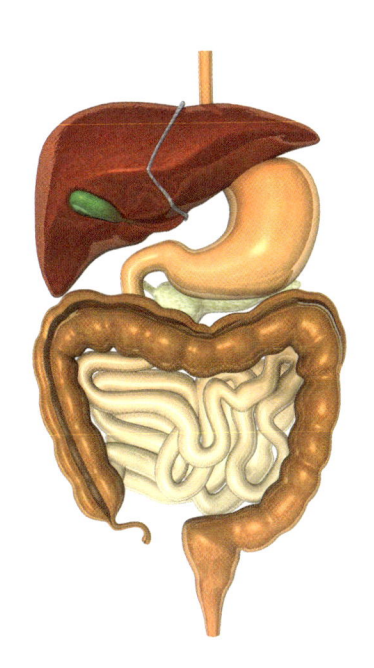

Name _____ Date _____

THE DIGESTIVE SYSTEM

Laboratory Review Questions

1. What lines most of the digestive tract?

2. What enzyme is secreted in the mouth during the presence of starch?

3. What structures in the small intestine enhance absorption?

4. What is the term for food after it enters the oral cavity?

5. What are the accessory structures of the digestive system?

Abdominal Cavity and Digestive Organs

6. Describe the functions of the liver.

7. What is the purpose of brush border enzymes? Where are they found?

8. What nerve(s) innervate the tongue and list their functions?

9. Describe the four basic digestive processes.

10. List the components of the digestive system. Shortly describe their functions.

11. What processes are involved in the mucosal turnover of the stomach and the small intestines?

12. What are the functions of the liver? Are all of the liver functions involved in digestion? Why?

13. What is the role of each general factor that is involved in regulation of the digestive system's functions?

14. Describe the factors involved in each type of motility in the components of the digestive tract.

15. Describe how vomiting is accomplished. What factors may influence vomiting?

16. List the enzymes involved in breaking proteins. Where in the digestive system would you find them?

17. List the enzymes involved in breaking sugars. Where in the digestive system would you find them?

18. Some of the digestive enzymes are secreted in their inactive form. How are they activated?

19. Describe some of the specific absorptions occurring within each component of the digestive tract. Describe the absorptive mechanisms specifically developed for salt, water, carbohydrates, proteins and fats.

20. A 45 year old woman was having a surgery on her gallbladder. Can she survive without her gallbladder? Why? What is the function of the gallbladder?

21. Describe the waste products excreted in the feces.

22. What is borborygmi?

23. What do you think is the function of the vermiform appendix?

24. What is are haustrae? What is their function.

25. Is vitamin absorption a passive or an active process? Why?

26. Where can you find the crypts of Lieberkuhn? What are their functions?

27. Name some of the causes for malabsorption.

28. What is the function of enterokinase? Where in the digestive system is it usually secreted.

29. Describe what peptic ulcers are. Describe environmental factors contributing in the development of ulcers?

30. What is the function of goblet cells?

31. What is the function of chief cells?

32. What is the function of parietal cells?

THE LYMPHATIC SYSTEM

IDENTIFY AND LOCATE

__ Cervical lymph nodes
__ Axillary lymph nodes
__ Abdominal lymph nodes
__ Inguinal lymph nodes
__ Lymphatics of mammary glands
__ Lymphatics of upper limb
__ Lymphatics of lower limb
__ Cisterna chyli
__ Thoracic duct (left lymphatic)
__ Right lymphatic duct
__ Thymus
__ Spleen

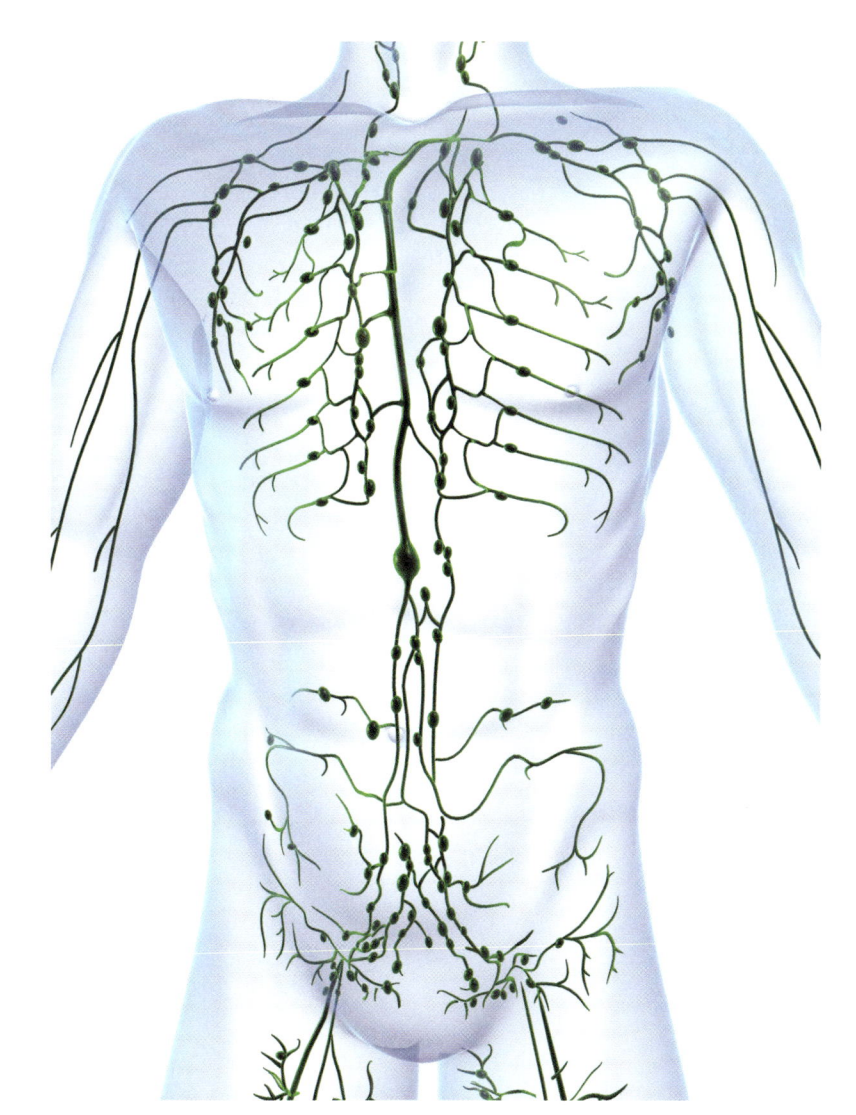

COMPONENTS OF LYMPHATIC SYSTEM

IDENTIFY AND LOCATE

__ Lymphatic vessel
__ Lymphatic valve
__ Collagen and elastic fibers

RELATIONSHIP OF LYMPHATIC DUCTS AND CIRCULATORY SYSTEM

IDENTIFY AND LOCATE

__ Thoracic duct
__ Right lymphatic duct
__ Left/right jugular trunks
__ Left/right subclavian trunks
__ Left/right internal jugular veins
   IDE

__ Left/right bronchomediastinal trunks
__ Left/right subclavian veins
__ Left/right brachiocephalic veins
__ Superior vena cava

IDENTIFY AND LOCATE

__ Gastrosplenic ligament
__ Superior/inferior borders
__ Diaphragmatic surface

__ Visceral surface   <Gastric area
                       <Renal area
__ Hilus (Splenic artery/vein)

IDENTIFY AND LOCATE

__ Connective tissue capsule
__ White pulp containing lymphocytes
__ Red pulp
__ Small trabecular arteries

Name _____ Date _____

THE LYMPHATIC SYSTEM
Laboratory Review Questions

1. What is the major role of the lymphatic system in the protection of our bodies?

   _____
   _____
   _____
   _____

2. Describe the shape of the spleen.

   _____
   _____
   _____
   _____

3. What is the name for the tonsils located on the posterior aspect of the tongue?

   _____
   _____
   _____
   _____

4. Where do lymphatic vessels originate?

   _____
   _____
   _____
   _____

5. What is/are the largest organ(s) of the lymphatic system? Describe the function(s).

   _____
   _____
   _____
   _____

6. Where can you find lymph nodes?

   _____
   _____
   _____
   _____

Abdominal Cavity and Digestive Organs

7. Name the components of the lymphatic system.

8. Why are there a large number of lymphatic vessels associated with the large intestine?

9. Describe the differences between innate and adaptive immunity.

10. What are the functions of the lymphoid tissues?

11. What are the differences between the classical and the alternative complement system?

12. Compare the maturations of the B cell and the T cells. Can you tell which ones are more effective? Why?

13. Define what an antigen is.

14. Define what an antibody is.

15. Define what the clonal theory is all about and how it exercises its effect? Be descriptive.

16. Define the function of macrophages.

17. Define the function of neutrophills.

18. If the thymus has been defective from birth, what impact would you expect it to have on the immune system of the child?

19. Describe the importance of class I and class II MHC glycoproteins.

20. Describe the mechanisms involved in developing tolerance in the immune system.

21. Define the differences between autoimmune disease and immune complex diseases.

22. What are the differences between immediate hypersensitivity and delayed hypersensitivity?

23. Describe some of the immune functions of the skin.

24. What is the function of the spleen?

25. What are the functions of membrane attack complexes (MAC)?

26. What is the role of thymosin?

27. What is an interferon?

28. List and describe the five classes of immunoglobulins.

29. What is anaphylactic shock?

30. What are the functions of helper T cells?

31. Define serum sickness.

32. Describe the differences between the primary and the secondary immune response.

33. What is opsonization?

The Male Reproductive System

Dissection of the Male Pelvic Organs

Required Instruments
Scalpel   Blade size 22   Retractors   Handles 3,4

1. Access the pelvic cavity by making a transverse incision along the superior margin of the pubic symphysis.

2. Deflect the rectus abdominus muscles laterally.

3. Explore the pelvic cavity to identify the urinary bladder, the ureters, and the ductus deferens.

4. Remove the tissue surrounding the ductus deferens along the inguinal ring after making an oblique incision following the inguinal canal.

5. Turn your attention to the sacral promontory and identify the major vessels: the common iliac artery and branches; the internal and external iliac arteries and veins.

6. At the level of the inguinal ligament, dissect superiorly to locate the femoral artery, vein, and nerve.

IDENTIFY AND LOCATE

__ Testis
__ Scrotum
__ Penis
__ Ductus deferens (vas deferens)

__ Spermatic cord
__ Seminal vesicle
__ Prostate gland
__ Bulbourethral gland

Observation of the Scrotum, Spermatic Cord, Testes, Epididymis, and Ductus Deferens

Testes

Spermatic Cord

Epididymis and Ductus Deferens

IDENTIFY AND LOCATE

__ Scrotum
__ Septa
__ Scrotal cavity
__ Lobules

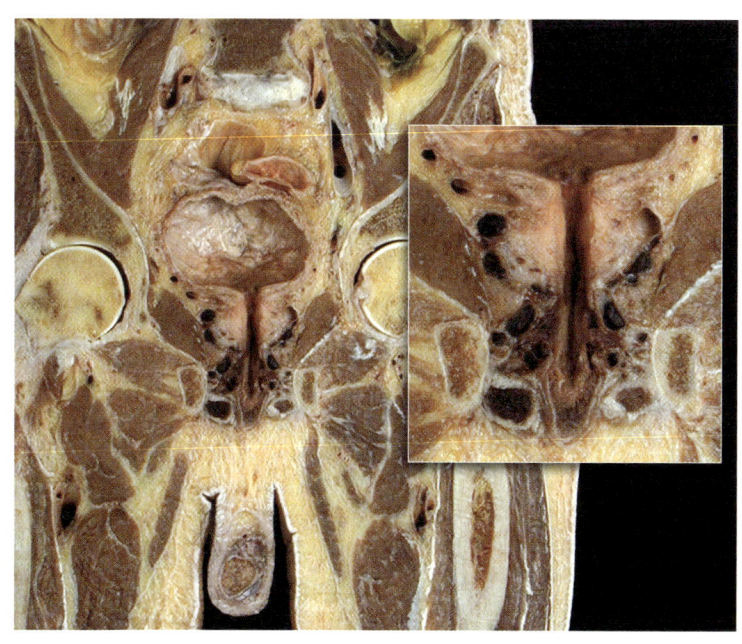

Photo by Mark Nielsen. Dissection by Shawn Miller.

Abdominal Cavity and Digestive Organs

__ Tunica vaginalis
__ Scrotal (Perineal) raphe
__ Testis
__ Tunica albuginea
__ Efferent ducts

__ Seminiferous tubules
__ Mediastinum
__ Straight tubules
__ Rete testis

__ Inguinal rings
__ Inguinal canal

           <Superficial
           <Deep

_Spermatic cord
           <External spermatic
           <fascia
           <Cremaster muscle/
           <fascia
           <Superficial scrotal
           <(dartos) fascia
           <Vas deferens
           <Arteries/Veins
           <Testicular
           <Pampiniform plexus
           <Inernal/external pudendal
           <Inferior epigastric

__ Epididymis
           <Head
           <Body
           <Tail

__ Ductus deferens
  (vas deferens)
           <Ampulla
           <Ejaculatory
           <duct

IDENTIFY AND LOCATE

__ Urinary bladder

__ Urethra segments
           <Prostatic
           <Membranous
           <Penile

__ Ductus deferens
__ Ejaculatory ducts
__ Seminal vesicles
__ Prostate gland
__ Bulbourethral glands

IDENTIFY AND LOCATE

__ General appearance of the gland
__ Pseudostratified columnar epithelium
__ Secretory pockets
__ Muscularis layer (smooth muscle fibers)
__ Adventitia

PROSTATE GLAND

IDENTIFY AND LOCATE

__ General appearance of the gland
__ Glands of the prostate (compound tubuloalveolar glands)
__ Smooth muscle/connective tissue

BULBOURETHRAL (COWPER'S) GLAND

IDENTIFY AND LOCATE

__ General appearance of gland
__ Mucous glands
__ Muscularis layer (smooth muscle fibers)
__ Connective tissue capsule

IDENTIFY AND LOCATE

__ Penis
  <Root (Crura and bulb)
  <Body (Shaft)
  <Glans

__ Corpora cavernosa
__ Corpus spongiosum

__ Urethra
  <Prostatic
  <Membranous
  <Penile

__ External urethral meatus
__ Prepuce
__ Dorsal blood vessels

__ Muscles
  <Ischiocavernous
  <Bulbocavernous

The Female Reproductive System

Observation of the Female Reproductive System

IDENTIFY AND LOCATE

__ Ovary
__ Uterine tube
__ Uterus
__ Vagina
__ Vesicouterine pouch
__ Rectouterine pouch

DISSECTION PROCEDURE

DISSECTION OF FEMALE REPRODUCTIVE ORGANS/UTERUS

Required Instruments
Scalpel   Blade size 22   Retractors   Handles 3,4

1. Make an incision along the superior margin of the pubic symphysis and deflect the abdominal muscles laterally.

2. Observe the organs of the pelvic cavity—the uterus, the broad ligament, and the fallopian tubes. Follow the length of the fallopian tubes to the end where the ovaries are located. Observe if there are several cysts or other abnormalities.

3. Palpate the uterus and observe its relationship to the urinary bladder and the rectum.

4. Make an incision on the uterine wall to expose the endometrium and observe the tissue structure.

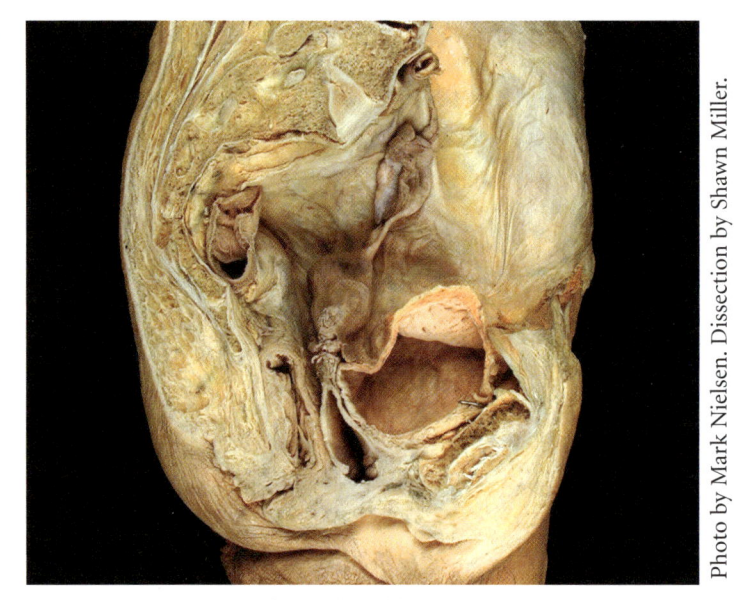

Observation of the Ovaries and Uterine Tubes

PELVIS MODULE

Photo by Mark Nielsen. Dissection by Shawn Miller.

THE UTERINE TUBES

IDENTIFY AND LOCATE

__ Ovary
__ Tunica albuginea
__ Broad ligament
__ Mesovarium
__ Suspensory ligament
__ Ovarian arteries/veins

__ Ovarian hilum
__ Ovarian ligament
__ Uterine tube
   <Infundibulum (Fimbriae)
   <Ampulla
   <Isthmus
   <Intramural

Observation of the Uterus and Vagina

IDENTIFY AND LOCATE

- __ Urinary bladder
- __ Uterus
  - \<Fundus
  - \<Body
  - \<Isthmus
  - \<Cervix
  - \<Uterine cavity
  - \<Cervical canal
  - \<External os

- __ Round ligaments of uterus
- __ Broad ligament
- __ Uterosacral ligaments
- __ Lateral (cardinal) ligaments
- __ Uterine arteries/veins

Internal Anatomy

- __ Uterine cavity
- __ Endometrium
- __ Myometrium
- __ Visceral peritoneum or serosal layer (Perimetrium)
- __ Cervix
- __ External os
- __ Cervical canal

Vagina

- __ Vaginal canal
- __ Fornix
- __ Vaginal rugae
- __ Vestibule
- __ Vaginal orifice

- __ Arteries/veins
  - \<Ovarian
  - \<Vaginal
  - \<Uterine

- __ Pudendal nerve

IDENTIFY AND LOCATE

- __ Uterine cavity
- __ Endometrium
  - \<Simple columnar
  - \<epithelium
  - \<Functional zone
  - \<Basilar zone
  - \<Endometrial glands

- __ Myometrium (Smooth muscle fibers)
- __ Perimetrium (Peritoneum)

Abdominal Cavity and Digestive Organs

IDENTIFY AND LOCATE

__ Mucosa layer <Stratified squamous <epithelium <(noncornified)

__ Muscularis (Smooth muscle fibers)
__ Adventitia

THE MAMMARY GLANDS

IDENTIFY AND LOCATE

__ Pectoralis major muscle
__ Pectoral fat pad
__ Suspensory ligaments
__ Mammary glands
__ Lactiferous ducts
__ Lactiferous sinus
__ Nipple
__ Areola

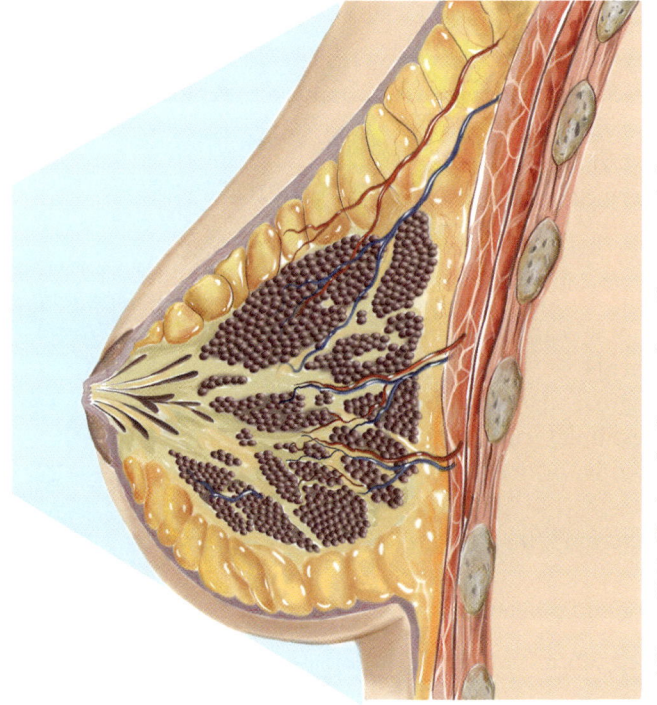

Name _____ Date _____

THE REPRODUCTIVE SYSTEM
Laboratory Review Questions

1. The body of the penis consists of what three masses?

2. The internal orifice connects the uterine cavity to which structure?

3. By what process are sperm cells produced?

4. What part of the spermatozoa contains the chromosomes?

5. What contains the ductus deferens, spermatic arteries/veins, nerves, and lymphatics that service the testes?

6. What are the finger-like projections of the infundibulim known as?

7. What is the layer of the uterus that provides mechanical protection and nutritional support for the developing embryo?

8. What is the inferior constricted portion of the uterus that projects into the vagina?

9. What is BPH? Is it a premalignant condition?

10. What is Crytorchidism? What does it result into?

11. What is the major hormone produced and secreted by the Leydig cells?

12. Why lactation doesn't happen during pregnancy?

13. Enumerate the effects of prolactin?

180   Abdominal Cavity and Digestive Organs

14. What is the best stimulant for lactation?

15. Where does fertilization usually occurs?

16. List some actions of testosterone, estrogen, and progesterone.

17. How is it possible that infections of the female reproductive system can spread to the abdominal cavity?

18. What is vasectomy?

19. What is tuball ligation?

20. What is the normal orientation of the uterus in relation to the vagina?

21. What is the "afterbirth"?

22. Name the hormone that triggers ovulation.

23. The first menstrual flow or period is known as _____.

24. What is oxytocin? How does it contribute to lactation?

25. The testes are the homologue structure of the female _____.

26. What hormones contribute to the LH surge?

27. Explain why there's variations in the length of menstrual cycle.

28. Explain the rationale behind oral contraceptives use.

The Urinary Organs

ORGANIZATION OF THE URINARY SYSTEM

The **urinary system** has many functions, including the formation of urine and the subsequent elimination of the organic waste products formed by body cells.

Other functions include: regulating blood volume and blood pressure; helping to maintain normal blood pH; stabilizing the plasma concentration of sodium, potassium, chloride, and calcium ions; and conserving valuable nutrients. The urinary system is the major regulator of ions and many of the organic molecules, like proteins, transported by the blood. Retaining or eliminating these substances is part of the work of the kidneys. The functions of the kidneys are indispensable to life. Other organs with excretory activities (skin, lungs, large intestine) cannot take over its functions. The urinary system consists of a pair of kidneys, a pair of ureters, a urinary bladder and a urethra. The urinary system is similar in men and women. The functions of the urinary system are exactly the same in both sexes, only the length and function of the structure (urethra) for the drainage of urine differ.

The **kidneys** are the organs of the urinary system, which remove waste products and stabilize both the volume and composition of the plasma. The modified, final waste product produced by the kidneys is termed **urine**. The kidneys are just as vital to life as the heart. Humans can survive either damage to one kidney or its removal but loss of both kidneys is life threatening. The bean-shaped kidneys lie of the posterior of the abdominopelvic cavity, between the dorsal body wall muscles and the parietal peritoneum. Since the kidneys are positioned behind the peritoneum, the term retroperitoneal is used to describe their location. Urine produced by the kidneys is transported though the **ureters**, a pair of muscular tubes that extend inferiorly from the kidneys, to a storage organ, the **urinary bladder**. It is held here until it can be eliminated from the body. The urinary bladder is located anterior to the rectum in the pelvic cavity. Urine is drained from the urinary bladder by a single tube, the **urethra**. In females the urethra is short and serves only to convey urine out of the body. In males the urethra is much longer, passing through the length of the penis. The urethra in males shares both excretory and reproductive functions.

IDENTIFY AND LOCATE

__ Right/left kidneys
__ Right/left ureters

__ Urinary bladder
__ Urethra (male and female)

IDENTIFY AND LOCATE

__ Renal capsule
__ Hilus
__ Renal artery/vein
__ Ureter
__ Cortex
__ Medulla
__ Renal pyramids
__ Renal columns

__ Renal sinus
__ Renal papillae
__ Renal pelvis
__ Major calyx
__ Minor calyx

IDENTIFY AND LOCATE

__ Abdominal aorta
__ Renal artery
__ Segmental arteries
__ Interlobar arteries
__ Arcuate arteries
__ Interlobular arteries
__ Afferent arterioles
__ Glomerulus
__ Efferent arterioles
__ Peritubular capillaries
__ Vasa recta capillaries
__ Interlobular veins
__ Arcuate veins
__ Interlobar veins
__ Segmental veins
__ Renal vein
__ Inferior vena cava

IDENTIFY AND LOCATE

__ Nephron

__ Renal corpuscle   <Glomerulus
                               <(Bowman's)
                               <capsule

__ Proximal convoluted tubule

                               <Descending limb
__ Loop of Henle   <Ascending limb
__ Distal convoluted tubule
__ Collecting tubule
__ Collecting duct

The Renal Corpuscle

__ Glomerulus
__ Capsular space
__ Capsular epithelium

                               <Afferent
__ Arterioles   <Efferent
__ Podocyte cells

Abdominal Cavity and Digestive Organs

IDENTIFY AND LOCATE

Cortical Region

__ Nephrons (cortical and juxtamedullary)
__ Renal corpuscle
__ Capsular space
__ Glomerulus
__ Capsular epithelium
__ Distal convoluted tubules
__ Proximal convoluted tubules

Medullary Region

__ Collecting duct
__ Capillaries

DISSECTION OF KIDNEYS

Required Instruments
Scalpel   Blade size 22   Retractors   Handles 3,4

1. After the abdominal cavity is opened and the abdominal viscera moved away from the site of incision of the posterior abdominal wall, make a longitudinal incision later to the cavity.
2. Extend your grasp to late the kidney and incise the perirenal fascia.
3. Carefully lifting the kidney, remove the surrounding fat and expose the hilum.
4. Preserve the adrenal glands that are positioned on the superior poles of the kidneys.
5. Remove the kidney after carefully identifying and incising the renal artery and vein. Leave a 2-3 margin of the uterter and incise to remove the kidney for further dissection on a tray.
6. You may leave one of the kidneys on the cadaver for further exploration and perception of organ relationships.
7. Continue dissection to identify the vessels providing blood to the adrenals.

URETHRA

IDENTIFY AND LOCATE

__ Peritoneum
__ Ureter
__ Urinary bladder
__ Rugae
__ Ureteral openings
__ Sphincter vesicae (internal urethral sphincter)

__ Trigone
__ Median umbilical ligament (urachus)
__ Lateral umbilical ligaments
__ Female urethra
__ External urethral meatus
                                    <Prostatic region
__ Male urethra   <Penile region
__ Sphincter urethrae (external sphincter) in urogenital diaphragm

IDENTIFY AND LOCATE

__ Lumen of ureter
__ Mucosa of transitional
    epithelium
      <Longitudinal
      <Smooth
      <(inner layer)
__ Muscularis
      <muscle
      <Circular
      <(outer) layer
__ Adventitia

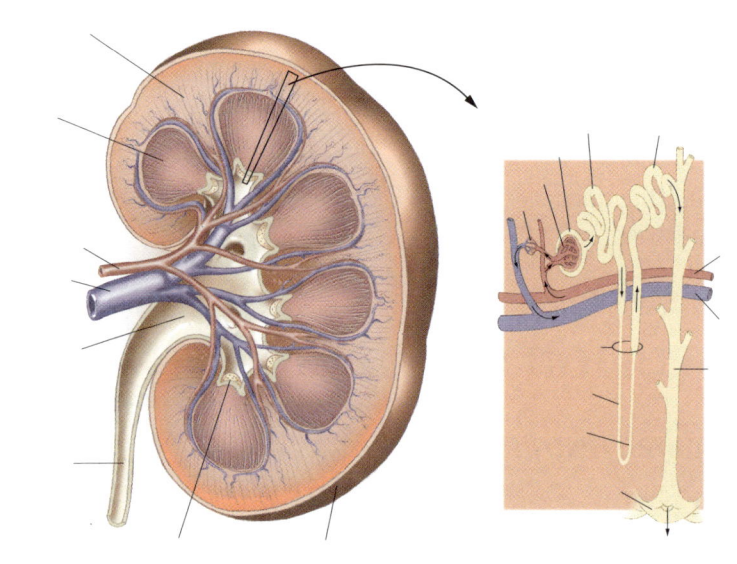

KIDNEY SECTIONAL VIEW

IDENTIFY AND LOCATE

__ Lumen of urinary bladder
                    <Transitional epithelium
__ Mucosa   <Lamina propria
__ Submucosa

                    <Detrusor muscle
                    <Longitudinal
                    <Smooth   <(inner) and (outer)
__ Muscularis   <muscle   <layers
                                  <Circular (middle)
                                  <layer

__ Serosa (Visceral peritoneum)
    (visible only on superior surface)

IDENTIFY AND LOCATE

__ Lumen of urethra

__ Mucosa   <Various epithelial types
                 <Lamina propria containing
                 <mucous epithelial glands

__ Muscularis   <Smooth   <Longitudinal (inner) layer
                   <muscle   <Circular (outer) layer

__ Serosa

DISSECTION OF THE PERINIUM

Required Instruments
Scalpel   Blade size 22   Saw   Blade size 10   Retractors   Handles 3,4

1. The perineum connects the vaginal orifice to the anus in females and the base of the scrotum to the anus in males.

2. The pelvic diaphragm containing the levetor ani and coccygeal muscles acts as a border between the perineum and the pelvic cavity.

3. In the female perineum, remember that one of the methods of episiotomy follows the perineal line.

4. In males, the prostate gland may be accessed through the perineum.

5. If the skin is removed by abducting the legs wider, the inferior boundary of the superficial perineal pouch can be identified after separating the superficial fascia from collis fascia.

6. Continue to identify the urogenital triangle.

7. Continue dissection to identify the pudendal nerve and artery in the deep perineal pouch.

8. In the female cadaver, identify the clitoris superior to the vaginal orifice and continue to dissect to expose the dorsal nerve and artery, which branch from the pudendal nerve and artery.

Name _____ Date _____

THE URINARY SYSTEM
Laboratory Review Questions

1. The renal medulla consists of six to eighteen distinct conical or triangular structures. What are they called?

   _____
   _____
   _____
   _____

2. The renal arteries give rise to the _____ arteries, which give rise to the interlobar arteries.

   _____
   _____
   _____
   _____

3. The triangular area bounded by the urethral openings and the entrance to the urethra constitutes what structure?

   _____
   _____
   _____
   _____

4. Kidneys are often difficult to see without dissection because they are surrounded by a layer of fat. What is the significance of this fat?

   _____
   _____
   _____
   _____

5. What is the expanded beginning of the ureter?

   _____
   _____
   _____
   _____

6. The urinary system interacts most closely with components of what other system?

7. The urinary bladder, ureters, and kidneys are located which way anatomically?

8. What is the structure that stores urine in the urinary tract?

THE URINARY SYSTEM: RENAL

Laboratory Review Questions

1. What does the term countercurrent (CC) refer to?

2. What does multiplier refer to?

3. The ECF deep in the medulla is 4 times saltier than the ECF near the _____.

4. What is the mOsm value of solute as it enters the DCT?

5. What happens as blood flows upward in the vasa recta?

6. Where are the JG cells located?

7. List the proper order of blood vessels that carry blood to the kidney.

8. Sympathetic stimulation of the kidney can accomplish _____

9. What is cotransport?

10. Peter has advanced arteriosclerosis. His blood values indicate elevated levels od aldosterone and decreased levels of ADH. Why?

11. What is the best indicator of renal function?

12. What is the normal level of creatinine in the body?

13. What percentage of cardiac output goes to the kidneys?

14. What do you NOT want to see in a urinalysis?

15. As far as endocrine function goes, the kidney regulates what 3 systemic parameters?

16. What are the usual symptoms of cystitis?

17. Angiotension II causes the adrenal gland to release what?

18. What hormone controls the FINAL concentration of urine?

19. What are normal specific gravity levels of urine?

20. What is tubular secretion?

21. What are the functions of the three forces involved in glomerular filtration?

22. What is the tubular maximum (TM)?

23. What limits of glucose reabsorption?

24. What is the renal threshold?

25. What structure monitors rate of flow through the distal tubule?

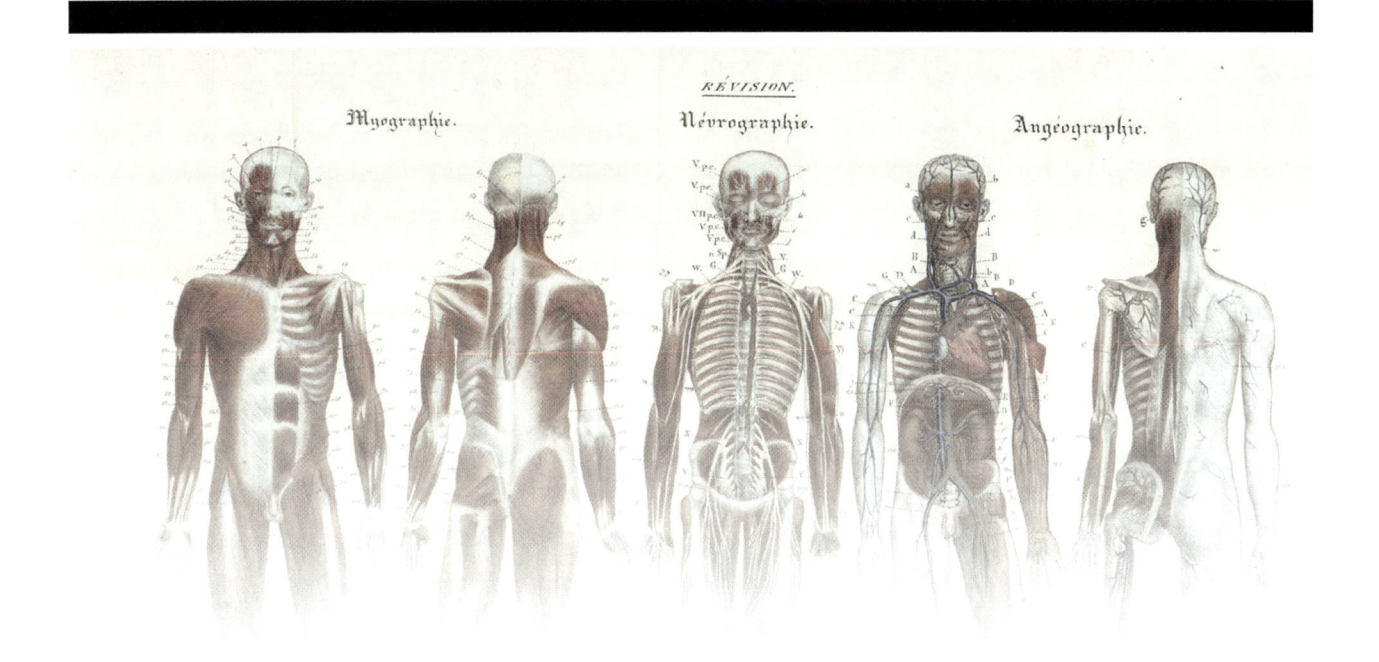

ENDOCRINE ORGANS

Observation of the Pituitary Gland (Hypophysis)

The pituitary gland or hypophysis is a small, pea-size gland that lies cradled within the sella turica of the sphenoid bone and is held in this protected position by the diaphragma sellae. The gland lies inferior to the hypothalamus, but is connected to it by a stalk, the infundibulum, which is encircled by the diaphragma sellae. Blood is supplied to the gland through the inferior hypophyseal artery. Anatomically, the pituitary gland is divided into posterior and anterior regions. It releases nine hormones (growth hormone, thyroid-stimulating hormone, adrenocorticotropic hormone, follicle-stimulating hormone, luteinizing hormone, prolactin, melanocyte-stimulating hormone, antidiuretic hormone, and oxytocin), many of which influence other endocrine glands. Please review the pituitary hormones and their targets prior to discussion.

Dissection Procedure

PREPARATION

Before you begin to identify the hypophysis (pituitary gland), review the sella turica of the sphenoid bone in a dry skull specimen and the landmarks of the diencephalons, both in sagittal section and on the intact brain.

Observation of the Pituitary Gland (Hypophysis)

Locate and identify the landmarks of the diencephalons (forebrain), using a torso head, a brain model, and specimen of the midbrain. Examine the landmarks of the diecephalon on the torso head model first. Observe the brain within the cranial cavity in sagittal section. Identify the optic chaism, mamillary body, median eminence, and the sella turcica of the sphenoid bone. Now locate the optic chiasm and mamillay bodies on the inferior surface of an intact brain model. Between these two landmarks, identify the infundibulum and the pituitary gland (hypophysis). The anterior lobe is that region of the pituitary gland anterior to the infundibulum, and the posterior lobe is the region that is connected directly to the infundibulum. In our next oberservation, we will use the microscope to identify cells in the major regions of these lobes. These regions can be observed only with the microscope. From the sagittal view, notice the location of the pituitary gland within the sella turcica of the sphenoid bone and its connection via the infundibulum to the hypothalamus.

IDENTIFY AND LOCATE

__ Sella turcica of sphenoid
__ Optic chiasma
__ Third ventricle
__ Median eminence
__ Mamillary body
__ Infundibulum
__ Pituitary gland
__ Posterior pituitary (Pars nervosa)

__ Anterior pituitary (Pars intermedia)
__ Anterior pituitary (Pars distalis)
__ Anterior pituitary (Pars tuberalis)

IDENTIFY AND LOCATE

__ Pars distalis
 (Anterior pituitary)
__ Pars intermedia
 (Anterior pituitary)
__ Pars nervosa
 (Posterior pituitary)

Observation of Thyroid Gland

The thyroid gland lies on the anterior and lateral surfaces of the trachea at the inferior region of the larynx (cricoid cartilage). The lateral surfaces of the gland are partially covered by the sternocleidomastoid, omohyoid, sternothyroid, and sternohyoid muscles. Thyroid follicles are simple cuboidal epithelial structures that surround the colloid-filled space termed the follicular cavity. They manufacture, store, and secrete the thyroid hormones, T3 (triiodothyronine) and T4 (thyroxin). Both speed up the rate of cellular metabolism and increase the use of oxygen by cells. The hormone calcitonin is produced and released by the C cells (parafollicular cells) in the thyroid and functions in the regulation of calcium ion concentration in body fluids. The thyroid removes iodine from the blood, then concentrates and stores it in the follicular cavity for later incorporation into thyroid hormones. An extensive blood supply to the gland provides quick access for these hormones to enter the bloodstream. Please review the targets and effects of the thyroid hormones prior to discussion.

Dissection Procedure

PREPARATION

Before you begin to examine the thyroid gland, review the anterior muscles of the neck: sternocleidomastoid, omohyoid, sternothyroid, and sternohyoid muscles.

Observe and identify the gross anatomy and surface of the thyroid gland, using the torso and a model or specimen of the thyroid gland. Using one of the aforementioned for reference, examine the thyroid gland located on the anterior and lateral surfaces of the trachea. Identify the superior border of the gland at the inferior portion of the larynx (thyroid and cricoid cartilages) and the inferior border of the gland at the second and third cartilage rings of the trachea. The thyroid gland has a "butterfly-like" appearance and consists of two lobes. Note both lobes of the thyroid gland as they curve around the cartilage rings. Observe that the two lobes are connected by a slender ribbon of tissue, the isthmus, at the level of the second or third tracheal rings. A capsule of connective tissue binds the gland to the trachea, but it is not present on models. Blood is supplied to the gland from two sources. Identify the superior thyroid artery, which is a branch of the external carotid artery, and the inferior thyroid artery, a branch of the thyrocervical trunk, Blood is drained from the gland by three veins. Locate and identify the superior and middle thyroid veins, which terminate in the internal jugular vein, and the inferior thyroid veins, which end at the brachiocephalic veins.

Use this description also to observe the thyroid glands in the cadaver. Observation of the thyroid gland in the cadaver requires retraction of both the sternocleidomastoid and omohyoid muscles. Each lobe of the thyroid can be observed as a dark brown, wedge-shaped structure. Examine the posterior surface of each lobe and note the convex shape. This shape permits its close attachment to the trachea. It is not always possible to identify all of the arteries and veins that service the thyroid.

IDENTIFY AND LOCATE

- __ Hyoid bone
- __ Larynx <Thyroid cartilage
          <Cricoid cartilage
- __ Trachea
- __ Right and left lateral lobes of thyroid gland
- __ Isthmus of thyroid gland
- __ Internal jugular vein

- __ Thyroid veins <Superior
                    <Middle
                    <Inferior
- __ Brachiocephalic vein
- __ Common carotid artery
- __ Thyroid arteries <Superior
                       <Inferior

IDENTIFY AND LOCATE

- __ Capsule of connective tissue
- __ C cells (parafollicular cells)
- __ Thyroid follicle
- __ Follicular cells
- __ Follicular cavity filled with colloid containing stored thyroglobulin

Endocrine Organs

Observation of the Parathyroid Glands

The four nodules that compose the parathyroid glands are atttached to the external, posterior surface of the thyroid gland by the thyroid capsule. These glands secrete parathormone (PTH), which regulates body fluid calcium ion concentration by opposing the effects of calcitonin. PTH is released when circulating calcium ion concentrations drop below normal. The level of blood calcium is increased by preventing its loss by kidney excretion, by removing it from storage in the bones, and by increasing its absorption across the digestive tract. A summary of the targets and effects of PTH are presented in Table 3.

Dissection Procedure

Locate and identify the groos anatomy and surgace features of the parathyroid gland, using the torso and a model or specimen of the parathyroid glands. Use one of the aforementioned for reference to observe the four pea-sized (nodules) parathyroid glands on the posterior surface of the thyroid lobes. On each lobe, identify both a superior and an inferior parathyroid gland nodule. The superior glands are located at the level of the first tracheal ring and the inferior glands are located at the level of the third tracheal ring, within the inferior portion of each thyroid gland, but do not surround them. This is not shown on models. Blood is supplied to the superior parathyroid glands by branches of the superior thyroid artery and to the inferior glands by branches of the inferior thyroid artery.

Use this description to observe also the parathyroid glands in the cadaver. Examine the posterior surface of both the right and left lobes of the thyroid. The connective tissue capsule of the thyroid serves not only to connect the parathyroid glands to the thyroid, but also, in most individuals, it separates the two glands. Occasionally the parathyroid glands are embedded within the tissue of the thyroid. In such cases you will not be able to observe these glands.

IDENTIFY AND LOCATE

__ Thyroid gland
__ Connective tissue capsule of parathyroid gland
__ Parathyroid glands (total of 2-superior and 2-inferior)

IDENTIFY AND LOCATE

__ Connective tissue capsule of parathyroid gland
__ Principal (chief) cells

Observation of the Adrenal (Suprarenal) Gland

The adrenal (suprarenal) glands lie on and cover the superior borders of the kidneys. Structurally and functionally, the adrenal glands are divided into two regions: a superficial adrenal cortex and an internal adrenal medulla. The cortex is subdivided into three regions or zona: (1) the outer zona glomerulosa, (2) the middle zona fasciculate, and (3) the inner zona reticularis. Each region produces different steroid hormones. The zona glomerulosa produces a collection of hormones termed the mineralocorticoid group, with aldosterone being the most significant of this group. The zona fasciculate produces a collection of hormones termed the glucocorticoids, with cortisone and cortisol being the most notable of this group. The zona reticularis is an additional source of sex hormones, both estrogen and androgens.

The inner core of the gland is the adrenal medulla, which produces both adrenaline (epinephrine) and noradrenalin (norepinephrine). The medulla is surrounded by and in contact with the zona reticularis of the cortex. Like the other endocrine glands, the adrenal glands are highly vascularized, with blood being supplied directly to the medulla first and then emanating out to the cortex. A summary of the targets and effects of the adrenal hormones is presented in Table 4.

Dissection Procedure

PREPARATION

Before you begin to observe the adrenal glands, review the abdominopelvic regions and viscera. Focus your attention on the lumbar and umbilical regions.

Locate the following adrenal gland structures using a torso and a model or specimen of the adrenal gland. To observe the adrenal glands clearly, remove all of the abdominopelvic viscera from the torso. Examine both the right and left lumbar regions and identify the brown bean-shaped kidneys. Identify the pyramid-shaped adrenal (suprarenal) glands that adhere to the superior and slightly medial surface of each kidney. Each gland is wrapped in a dense, fibrous connective tissue capsule, which binds the gland to the kidney and separates the two structures. Located medial to each adrenal gland and projecting along the posterior abdominal wall are the two major blood vessels, the abdominal aorta supplying blood to all of the abdominopelvic structures and lower extremities, and the inferior vena cava draining blood from these regions back to the heart. Identify the blood supply both to the kidneys and to the adrenal glands. The renal arteries, which are major branches of the aorta, supply blood to each kidney. Identify branches of the renal arteries, the inferior suprarenal arteries, which supply blood to the inferior portions of the adrenal glands. Superior to the renal arteries, identify the middle suprarenal arteries and the superior suprarenal arteries. Both of these branches supply blood to the remainder of the glands. Blood is drained from the adrenals by the suprarenal veins.

Observe the adrenal gland in sectional view to examine its regions. From the exterior inward, identify the connective tissue capsule that surrounds the gland. Immediately under the connective tissue layer, identify the thick adrenal cortex. Deep to the cortex, the highly vascularized inner core, the adrenal medulla, is completely surrounded by cortex.

Use the description provided to observe the adrenal glands in the cadaver.

IDENTIFY AND LOCATE

__ Kidneys
__ Adrenal glands
__ Cortex
__ Medulla
__ Renal arteries
__ Renal veins
__ Superior suprarenal arteries
__ Middle suprarenal arteries
__ Inferior suprarenal arteries
__ Suprarenal veins

IDENTIFY AND LOCATE

__ Adrenal gland
          <Zona glomerulus
__ Cortex<Zona fasciculate
          <Zona reticularis
__ Medulla

Name _____ Date _____

THE ENDOCRINE SYSTEM
Laboratory Review Questions

1. In general, what are the effects of the nervous system?

2. The anterior pituitary can be divided into what two regions?

3. The alpha cells of the pancreas produce what hormone?

4. What are the blood vessels that supply or drain the thyroid gland?

5. List the reasons why the adrenal medulla is difficult to establish as either a nervous or an endocrine system structure.

6. What are peripheral cells sensitive to the presence of hormones called?

7. The zona glomerulosa of the adrenal gland produces what hormones?

8. How does aging affect the function of the endocrine system?

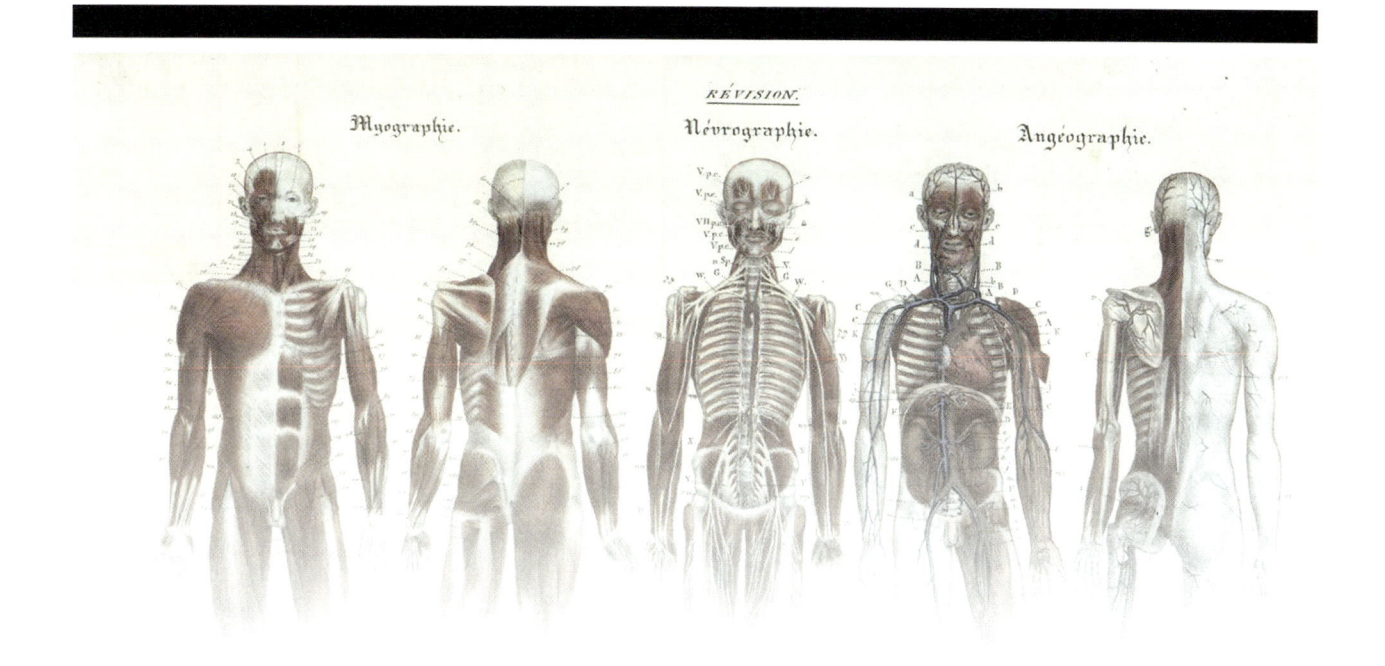

NERVOUS SYSTEM ORGANS AND STRUCTURES

Observations of the General Senses of the Skin

IDENTIFY AND LOCATE

__Nasal conchae (turbinates)
__Cribriform plate
__Crista galli
__Olfactory epithelium
__Olfactory bulb
__Olfactory tract

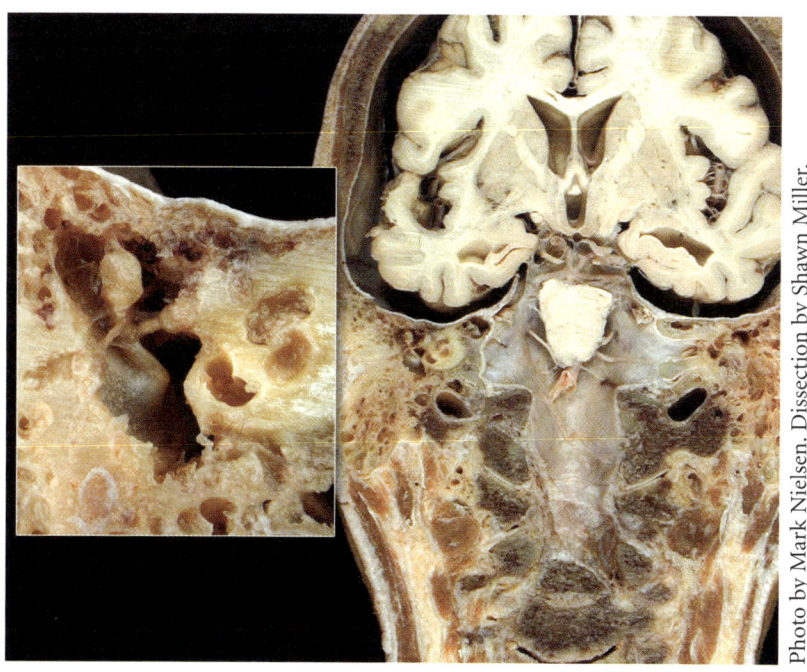

IDENTIFY AND LOCATE

__Olfactory epithelium
__Olfactory receptor cells
__Supporting cells
__Olfactory (Bowman's) gland

Observation of the Tongue

IDENTIFY AND LOCATE

__Dorsal surface (dorsum) of tongue
__Distribution of papillae   <Filiform
  <Fungiform
  <Circumvallate

Observation of Cranial Nerves of Gustation

IDENTIFY AND LOCATE

__Facial (N VII)
__Glossopharyngeal (N IX)
__Vagus (N X)

IDENTIFY AND LOCATE

__Papillae <Filiform
  <Fungiform
  <Circumvallate
__Taste buds
__Gustatory cell
__Supporting cell
__Taste pore
__Microvilli (taste buds)

Name _____ Date _____

THE NERVOUS SYSTEM: GENERAL AND SPECIAL SENSES

Laboratory Review Questions

1. What is a sensory receptor?

2. Which cranial nerves transmit sensory information from the taste buds?

3. What are the three main regions of the ear?

4. How many auditory ossicles are there? What are their names? How did they receive their names?

5. The place where the two optic nerves reach the diencephalons is called?

6. Name the structures of the external ear from the outside to the inside.

7. What happens when someone contracts "pink eye," and what is its medical name?

8. What is the function of the structures within the middle ear?

The Brain and Cranial Nerves

Organization of the Brain: Major Regions and Landmarks

Dissection Procedure

PREPARATION

In light of the time frame for the semsester, individual nerve dissection is not practically feasible at NSC. The meninges and the major parts of the brain, however, can be observed after craniotomy.

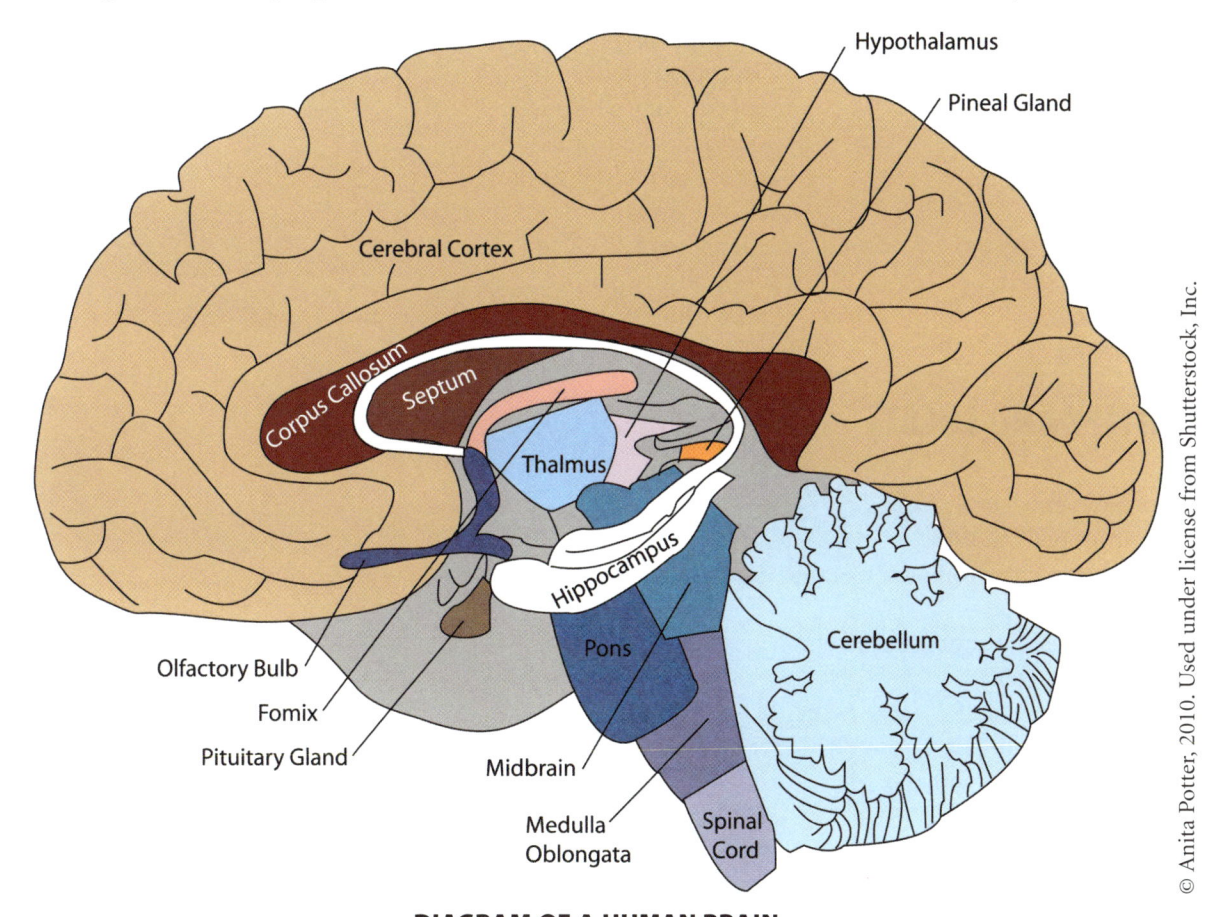

DIAGRAM OF A HUMAN BRAIN

IDENTIFY AND LOCATE

Overview of the Brain

__Cerebrum (right/left cerebral hemispheres)
__Longitudinal tissue
__Cerebellum
__Pons
__Medulla oblongata

__Telencephalon (cerebrum)
__Diencephalon (hypothalamus and thalamus)
__Mesencephalon (midbrain)
__Metencephalon (cerebellum & pons)
__Myelencephalon (medulla oblongata)

IDENTIFY AND LOCATE

__Cranial meninges
    <Dura mater
    <Arachnoid
    <Pia mater
__Cerebral hemispheres
__Cerebellum/medulla oblongata/spinal cord
__Dura mater
(connects at four locations in the cranial
    <Falx cerebri
    <Tentorium cerebelli
    <Falx cerebelli
    <Diaphragma sellae
__Sinuses within the dura mater
    <Superior sagittal sinus
    <Inferior sagittal sinus
    <Transverse sagittal sinus
    <Straight sinus
__Structures and spaces of the arachnoid
    <Arachnoid trabeculae
    <Subdural space
    <Subarachnoid space
__Pia mater

IDENTIFY AND LOCATE

__Lateral ventricles (1st and 2nd)
__Septum pellucidum
__Interventricular foramen (foramen of Monro)
__Third ventricle
__Mesencephalic aqueduct (cerebral aqueduct)
__Fourth ventricle
__Choroid plexus of 4th ventricle
__Lateral/median apertures of 4th ventricle
__Central canal of spinal cord
__Subarachnoid space

IDENTIFY AND LOCATE

__Cerebral hemisphere (left/right)
__Sulci
    <Central
    <Lateral
    <Parieto-occipital
    <(Note: locate
    <from medial view)
__Longitudinal fissure

__Cerebral lobes
    <Frontal
    <Temporal
    <Parietal
    <Occipital
__Insula   <(Deep in lateral fissure)
__Gyri
    <Precentral
    <Postcentral

IDENTIFY AND LOCATE

__Lobes
    <Frontal
    <Parietal
    <Temporal
    <Occipital

__Cortex
    <Primary motor (precentral gyrus)
    <Visual
    <Auditory
    <Olfactory
    <Primary sensory (postcentral gyrus)

__Sulci
    <Central
    <Lateral
    <Parieto-occipital

__Association areas
    <Somatic motor (premotor cortex)
    <Visual association
    <Auditory association
    <Sensory association

IDENTIFY AND LOCATE

__Central white matter
    <Association fibers
    <Commissural fibers
    <Projection fibers

__Commissural fibers
    <Corpus callosum
    <Anterior commissure

__Association fibers
    <Arcuate fibers
    <Longitudinal fasciculi

__Projection fibers
    <Internal capsule

IDENTIFY AND LOCATE

__Corpus striatum
    <Caudate nucleus
    <Lentiform nucleus
        <Putamen
        <Globus pallidus

__Claustrum
__Amygdaloid body

Observation of the Limbic System

IDENTIFY AND LOCATE

__Limbic lobe
    <Cingulate gyrus
    <Parahippocampal gyrus

__Temporal lobe
__Corpus callosum
__Hippocampus
__Fornix
__Mamillary body

IDENTIFY AND LOCATE

__Epithalamus
__Pineal gland
__Thalamus (walls of the diencephalons surrounding the 3rd ventricle)
__Interthalmic adhesion

__Optic chiasma
__Infundibulum
__Hypothalamus   <Tuber cinereum
  (floor of the   <Paraventricular nucleus
  3rd ventricle)   <Supraoptic nucleus
                           <Preoptic area

IDENTIFY AND LOCATE

__Thalamus
__Tectum   <Superior colliculus
  (roof)   <Inferior colliculus
__Corpora quadrigemina

__Wall and   <Red nucleus
  floor   <Substantia nigra
  structures
__Cerebral peduncles

Observation of the Metencephalon (Cerebellum and Pons)

IDENTIFY AND LOCATE

Cerebellum

__Folia
__Lobes   <Anterior
        <Posterior
        <Flocculonodular
__Primary fissure
__Vermis
__Cerebellar hemispheres
__Cerebellar cortex
__Arbor vitae

              <Superior
__Cerebellar   <Middle
  peduncles   <Inferior
__Medulla oblongata
__Choroid plexus of 4th ventricle

Pons
__Gray matter
__White matter

IDENTIFY AND LOCATE

__Pons
__Medulla oblongata
__Spinal cord
__Olives
__Olivary nuclei

__Nucleus gracilis
__Nucleus cuneatus
__Nuclei of   <N VIII, N IX
  cranial nerves   <N X, N XI, N XII

Observation of the Cranial Nerves

LOCATE

__Cerebrum
                                 <Olfactory nerve fibers
__Olfactory nerve (N I)   <Olfactory bulb
  (Passes through   <Olfactory tract
   cribiform plate)
__Diencephalon
__Optic nerve (N II)   <Optic tracts
  (Passes through   <Optic chiasma
   optic canal)
__Mesencephalon
__Oculomotor nerve (N III) {Ciliary ganglion
  (Passes through superior orbital fissure)
__Trochlear nerve (N IV)
  (Passes through superior orbital fissure)
__Pons
                               <Branches
__Trigeminal   <Semilunar (trigeminal) ganglion
   nerve (N V)   <Ophthalmic (Passes through superior orbital fissure)
   and branches   <Maxillary (Passes through foramen rotundum)
                               <Mandibular (Passes through foramen ovale)
__Abducens nerve (N VI)
  (Passes through superior orbital fissure)
                               <Geniculate ganglion
__Facial nerve (N VII)   <Petropalatine ganglion
   and associated   <Submandibular ganglion
   ganglia (Passes
   through internal
   acoustic meatus to stylomastoid foramen)
                               <Branches
__Vestibulocochlear nerve   <Vestibular nerve
   (N VIII)   <Cochlear nerve
   (Passes through internal
    acoustic meatus)
                               <Ganglia
__Glossopharyngeal nerve <Superior ganglion
   (N IX)   <Inferior (petrosol)
   (Passes through   <ganglion
    jugular foramen)

                               <Ganglia
                               <Superior (jugular) ganglion
                               <Inferior (nodose) ganglion

__Vagus nerve (N X)
(passes through
 jugular foramen)

<Nerve branches
<Superior laryngeal
<Internal laryngeal
<External laryngeal
<Recurrent laryngeal nerve
<Cardiac nerves

<Branches
__Accessory nerve (N XI) <Medullary (cranial)
(Passes through jugular <Spinal
 foramen)

__Hypoglossal nerve (N XII)
(Passes through hypoglossal canal)

Name _____ Date _____

THE NERVOUS SYSTEM: THE BRAIN AND CRANIAL NERVES
Laboratory Review Questions

1. What do the cranial blood vessels flow under?

2. What are the structures of the diencephalons?

3. What is the function(s) of the cerebellum?

4. What are the cranial nerves that move the eye?

5. What is the name for the groove between the frontal and parietal lobes of the brain?

6. Which nerve provides sensory information for taste on the anterior 2/3 of the tongue?

7. What are the functions of the cerebrospinal fluid?

8. What structures protect the brain against impact on the interior of the cranium?

THE NERVOUS SYSTEM: THE SPINAL CORD AND SPINAL NERVES

Gross Anatomy of the Spinal Cord, Spinal Nerves, and Spinal Meninges

IDENTIFY AND LOCATE

__Spinal cord emerging from foramen magnum of occipital bone
__The 31 pairs of spinal nerves
__Cervical spinal nerves (C1-C8)
__Cervical enlargement
__Thoracic spinal nerves (T1-T12)
__Lumbar spinal nerves (L1-L5)
__Lumbar enlargement
__Sacral spinal nerves (S1-S5) emerging from sacral foramina
__Cauda equina
__Filum terminale

Observation of the Spinal Cord, Spinal Nerves, and Meninges

IDENTIFY AND LOCATE

__Spinal cord

__Menininges   <Meninges
                   <Arachnoid
                   <Pia mater

__Spinal nerves

SECTIONAL ANATOMY OF THE SPINAL CORD: MICROSCOPIC IDENTIFICATION

IDENTIFY AND LOCATE

__Spinal cord
__Dura mater
__Arachnoid
__Pia mater
__Ventral root
__Gray matter
__White matter

__Anterior median fissure
__Posterior median sulcuc
__Central canal
__Dorsal root ganglion
__Dorsal root

__Gray horns   <Posterior
                <Anterior
                <Lateral

Nervous System Organs and Structures

IDENTIFY AND LOCATE

__Vertebral body
__Vertebral foramen
__Spinal cord
__Epidural space
__Dura mater

__Arachnoid
__Subarachnoid
__Pia mater
__Denticulate ligaments
__Ventral root

__Dorsal root ganglion
__Dorsal root
__Dorsal ramus
__Ventral ramus

IDENTIFY AND LOCATE

__Cervical spinal nerves (C1-C8)
__Nerve roots of Cervical plexus
   C1-C4: Ansa cervicalis complex
   C2-C3: Lesser occipital, transverse cervical, supraclavicular, and greater auricular nerves

C3-C5: Phrenic nerves
Cz-C5: Cervical nerves

IDENTIFY AND LOCATE

__Cervical spinal nerves (C5-C8)
__Thoracic spinal nerves (T1-T2)
__Nerve roots C5-T1 of Brachial plexus

__Brachial plexus
__Lateral cord
__Medial cord
__Posterior cord

<Superior trunk
<Middle trunk
<Inferior trunk
<Musculocutaneous nerve
<Lateral root of median nerve
<Medial root of median nerve
<Ulnar nerve
<Axillary nerve
<Radial nerve

IDENTIFY AND LOCATE

__Thoracic spinal nerves (T10-T12)
__Lumbar spinal nerves (L1-L5)
__Nerve roots T12-L4 of lumbar plexus
__Iliohypogastric nerve (L1)
__Ilioinguinal nerve (L1)
__Genitofemoral nerve (L1, L2)
__Lateral femoral cutaneous nerve (L1-L3)
__Femoral nerve (L2-L4)
__Obturator nerve (L2-L4)
__Saphenous nerve (L2-L4)

216   Nervous System Organs and Structures

IDENTIFY AND LOCATE

__Lumbar spinal nerves (L1-L5)
__Sacral spinal nerves (S1-S5) emerging from sacral foramina
__Nerve roots L4-S4 of sacral plexus
__Gluteal nerves   <Superior
  (L4-S2)   <Inferior
__Sciatic nerve   <Tibial branch
  (L4-S3)   <Common fibular branch
__Pudendal nerve (S2-S4)
__Lateral sural cutaneous nerve
__Medial sural cutaneous nerve
__Sural nerve

Name _____ Date _____

THE NERVOUS SYSTEM: THE SPINAL CORD AND SPINAL NERVES

Laboratory Review Questions

1. What are the components of the central nervous system (CNS)?

2. What is the function of the spinal meninges?

3. How many regions are there in the spinal cord? List them.

4. Are the meninges different for the brain and spinal cord? Explain.

5. Decribe the function and structure of the pia mater.

6. What is the name for the increased amount of grey matter in the lumbar region of the spinal cord?

7. What is the most common region of injury for a paraplegic?

8. What nerve(s) is/are associated in innervating the toes?

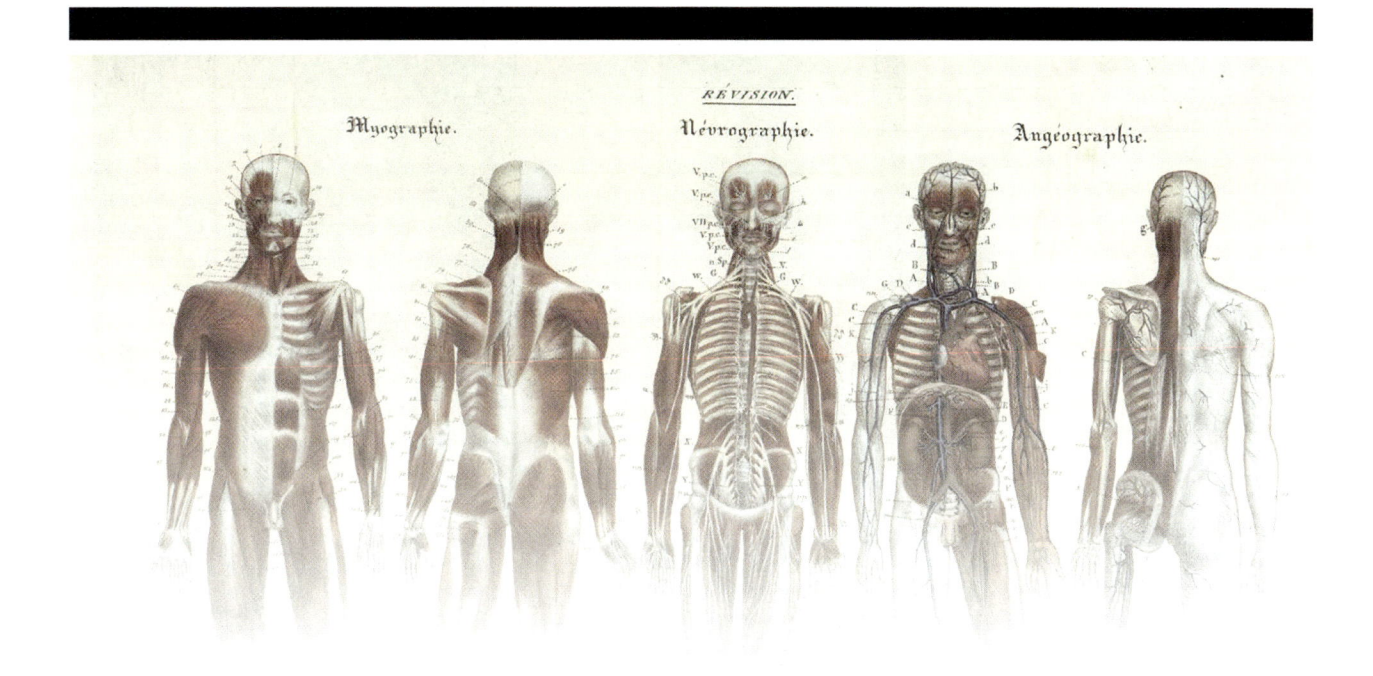

THE SENSORY ORGANS

Observation of Ear Anatomy

IDENTIFY AND LOCATE

__External, middle, and inner ear divisions
__Auricle
__External acoustic meatus
__Tympanic membrane (tympanum)
__Auditory ossicles
__Temporal bone (petrous portion)
__Auditory tube (pharyngotympanic tube or Eustachian tube)
__Bony labyrinth of inner ear
__Vestibular complex
__Cochles
__Vestibulocochlear   <Cochlear division
   (N VIII) nerve   <Vestibular division

IDENTIFY AND LOCATE

__External acoustic meatus
        <Malleus
__Auditory ossicles
        <Incus
        <Stapes
__Base of stapes in oval window
__Oval window
__Tensor tympani muscle
__Stapedius muscle
__Auditory tube

IDENTIFY AND LOCATE

__Cochlea
__Endolymphatic sac
__Vestibular complex
__Macula in saccule
__Bony labyrinth
__Membranous labyrinth

__Semicircular

__Ampullae (one for each duct)
__Utricle
__Saccule
__Endolymphatic duct

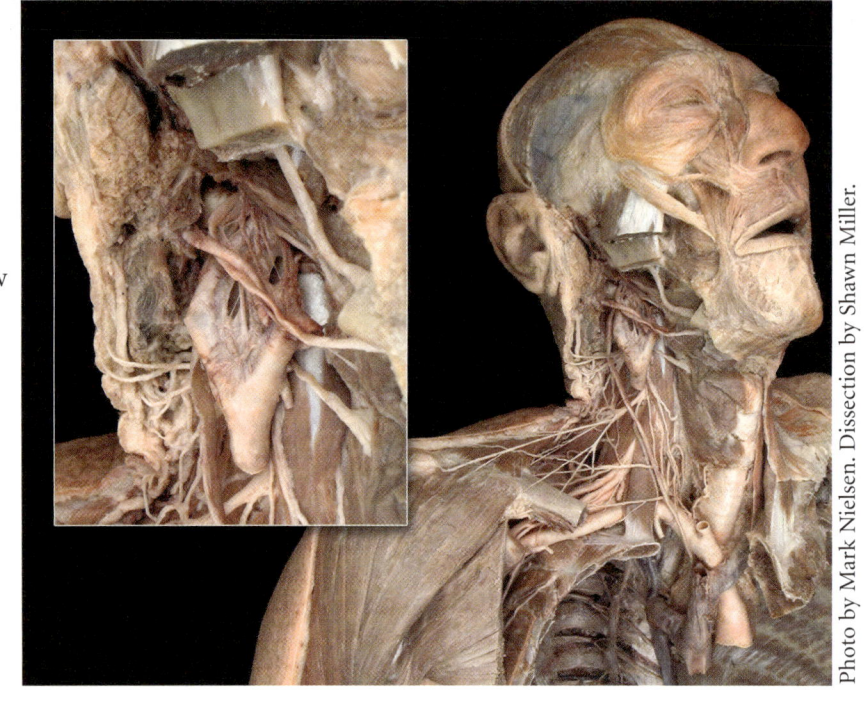

__Macula in utricle
    <Anterior
    <Posterior
    <Lateral

__Vestibular duct (scala vestibule)
__Cochlear duct (scala media)
__Tympanic duct (scala tympani)
__Round window
__Oval window

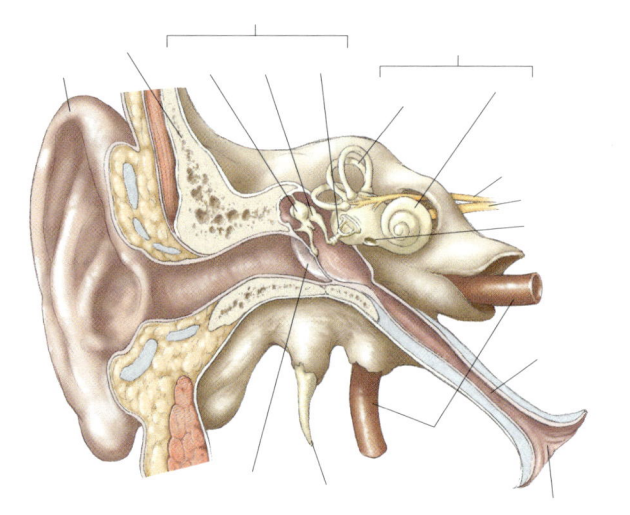

IDENTIFY AND LOCATE

__Vestibular duct (scala vestibule)
__Bony cochlear wall
__Cochlear duct (scala media)
__Tactorial membrane
__Organ of Corti
    <Basilar membrane
    <Hair cells

__Tympanic duct (scala tympani)
__Spiral ganglion of cochlear nerve
__Cochlear nerve
__Vestibulocochlear nerve (N VIII)

Observation of Accessory Structures of the Eye and Procedure

PREPARATION

Before you begin to examine the anatomy of the eye ball, stand in front of your lab partner and observe the eye and its accessory structures. Alternatively, you can use the diagrams and illustrations in your book as a guide.

Ask your lab partner to move their eyes superiorly, inferiorly, laterally, and medially. Ask them also to roll their eyes superiorly and inferiorly. These actions are accomplished by the muscles of the eye that are attached to the sclera, which is the outermost durable coat of the eye. Palpate the outer borders of the orbit gently and closely observe how the eye ball is contained in the orbital socket. Using a lighting pen observe the changes the pupil undergoes when you throw the light rays on it. This is referred to as pupilary dilation and constriction.

Since cadaveric eyes may not be ideal for dissection, you may use a specimen such as a bovine eye, and dissect on a tray.

You may locate the following structures on your lab partner and others on the specimen or on the cadaver. For a comprehensive understanding of these structures, it is beneficial to use all the resources available to you.

IDENTIFY AND LOCATE

__Palpebrae (Eyelids)
__Orbicularis oculi muscle
__Conjunctiva
__Eyelashes
__Palpebral fissure
__Medial canthus
__Lateral canthus
__Lacrimal caruncle
__Sclera
__Pupil

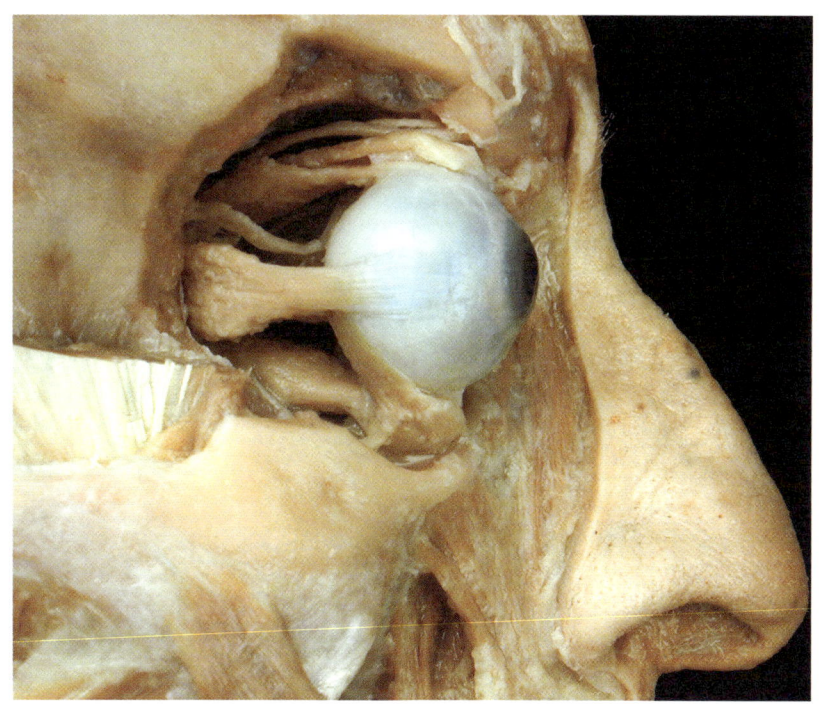

Photo by Mark Nielsen. Dissection by Shawn Miller.

ANATOMY OF THE ACCESSORY STRUCTURES: THE LACRIMAL APPARATUS

IDENTIFY AND LOCATE

__Upper/lower eyelids
__Lacrimal gland
__Lacrimal puncta
__Lacrimal canaliculi (ducts)
__Superior lacrimal canal

__Inferior lacrimal canal
__Lacrimal sac
__Nasolacrimal duct
__Opening of nasolacrimal duct

The Sensory Organs

Observation of the Extraocular Eye Muscles

IDENTIFY AND LOCATE

__Superior oblique muscle
__Superior rectus muscle
__Medial rectus muscle
__Trochlear nerve (IV)
__Oculomotor nerve (III)
__Abducens nerve (VI)
__Lateral rectus muscle

__Inferior rectus muscle
__Inferior oblique muscle

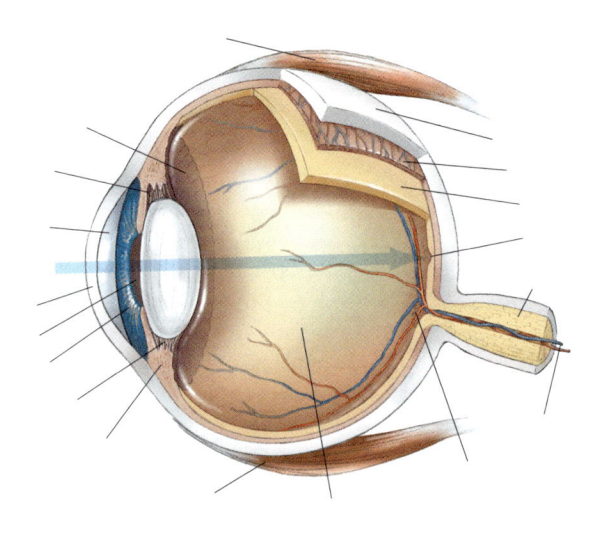

IDENTIFY AND LOCATE

Tunics (Layers) of the Eye

__Fibrous (sclera, cornea)
__Vascular (choroid, ciliary body, iris)
__Neural (retina)

Structures

__Conjunctiva
    <Ocular
    <Palpebral
__Fornix
__Sclera
__Cornea
__Limbus
__Anterior chamber
__Pupil
__Iris
__Ciliary body
__Ora serrata
__Lens
__Suspensory ligaments

__Posterior chamber
__Vitreous (humor) chamber/body
__Choroid
__Pigmented layer
__Retina
__Fovea (fovea centralis)
__Optic disc
__Optic nerve
__Central retinal artery
__Central retinal vein

IDENTIFY AND LOCATE

__Sclera
__Choroid
__Pigment layer of retina
__Photoreceptors
    <Rods
    <Cones
__Bipolar cells
__Ganglion cells
__Fovea
__Optic disc

Eye Dissection

Required Instruments
Scalpel   Blade size 22   Dissecting tray   Gloves   Paper towel

Identification of External Structure

Sclera
Cornea
Orbital fat
Extraocular muscles
    Superior rectus
    Medial rectus
    Inferior rectus
    Lateral rectus
    Superior oblique
    Inferior oblique
Conjunctiva
Optic nerve

Identification of Internal Structures

Iris
Pupil
Ciliary body
Lens
Zonule fibers
Angle of the eye
Posterior segment
Vitreous
Retina
Choroid
Optic nerve head
Optic nerve

Dry the eye and the dissecting pan with paper towels. With the globe held firmly and the globe not sliding around, place your blade 1-2 mm above the optic nerve and cut toward the cornea ensuring the blade is parallel to the table at all times. Once you've reach the lens, which will be difficult to cut through, turn the eye 90 degrees so the cornea is facing down on the dissecting pan without removing the blade from the eye. Once in position, apply firm pressure on the blade. Once you've cut through the lens, keeping the eye in the same position, carefully and gently cut through the iris and cornea.

1. Once you have removed the cap, the intraocular structures are readily visible. To better appreciate the globe's internal anatomy, it is best to approach the anatomy from the cornea to the optic nerve (i.e., anterior to posterior).

2. The cornea is fairly thick. Observe the thickness of the sclera, the junction between the cornea and the sclera (i.e., the limbus) and, posteriorly, the optic nerve. The cornea is the primary refractive index of the eye and important in bending light rays.

3. The middle layer, tunica vasculosa, is black and contains the iris (regulates the amount of light entering the eye), ciliary body (aqueous humor production, accommodation, and focusing), and choroid (nourishes the outer layers of the retina). In the anterior segment, the iris and ciliary body are homogenous in color. The choroid, which lies in the posterior segment, may be heterochromatic (i.e., region(s) black to blue-green or grayish), often referred to as the *tapetum lucidum*. This is due to the different degree of pigmentation of the choroid. The *tapetum lucidum* reflects light from the back of the eye. Keep in mind the *tatepum lucidum* is not present in human eyes but readily seen in lower animals (i.e., cat, cow, sheep).

4. The space bordered by the posterior surface of the cornea and the anterior surface of the iris is the anterior chamber.

5. The junction where the iris meets the limbus is the angle of the eye. You may be able to visualize the canal of Schlemm if viewed under a dissecting microscope. This is the point where aqueous humor is drained from the anterior chamber.

6. Posterior to the iris and medial to the ciliary body is the lens. Notice the fine, thin, delicate zonule fibers (suspensory ligaments) arising from the ciliary body and inserting on the posterior lens capsule. If you have difficulty seeing these fibers, gently lift the lens away from its anatomical position. You should feel resistance, and the "white" strands holding the lens are the zonule fibers. The ciliary body and zonule fibers are important in changing the shape of the lens allowing the image to properly focus on the retina.

7. Posterior to the lens is the vitreous humor. The vitreous is a gelatinous material that helps stabilize the globe and supports the retina. As a person ages, the vitreous takes on a more watery consistency, termed synersis (liquefication of the gel). This condition is one of the leading contributing factors to the development of a retinal detachment. As the vitreous gel begins to liquefy, the vitreous structure begins to pull toward the center, which in turn tugs on the retina. The pulling force and the shearing mechanism lead to a small tear in the retina that can ultimately lead to a larger retinal detachment that may lead to blindness if the macula is detached.

8. Located between the vitreous humor and the choroid (dark, bluish color) is a dull white structure—the retina. Anatomically, the retina has ten (10) layers. Functionally, the retina is divided into two layers: the outer pigmented epithelium termed the retinal pigment epithelium, and the inner neural layers, which is important in photochemistry and electrical conduction. The retina is best viewed under a microscope where the layers of retina are readily identifiable.

9. Examine closely and you will see at the most posterior region of the globe the retina "bundle" up. Correlating to the external posterior area, you will see that is where the optic nerve exits the eye. The optic nerve is a collection of ganglion cell axons. Its function is to convey the electrical impulses to the occipital lobe for visual image processing.

Name _____   Date _____

THE SPECIAL SENSE ORGANS: EAR AND EYE

Laboratory Review Questions

1. Name the chambers of the eye and list what is found in each chamber.

2. Describe the components of the retina and explain how each structure is related to its function.

3. Describe the formation and circulation of aqueous humor.

4. What is the clinical importance of the canal of Schlemm?

5. Describe the histological structure and organization of the inner ear.

6. Describe the path of sound waves entering the ear.

7. Outline the histological organization of the cochlear canal.

8. What do meibomian glands secrete and why? What is an inflammation of these ducts called?

Name _____ Date _____

THE SPECIAL SENSE ORGANS: EYE

Laboratory Review Questions

1. The two types of photoreceptors are _____ and _____. The _____ are predominantly located in the periphery of the _____ while the _____ are concentrated in the _____.

2. A near-sighted person is _____ while those that are far-sighted are _____.

3. The axons of the _____ cells project to the posterior of the eye, exiting the lamina cribosa giving rise to the _____ nerve.

4. Cataract, an age related condition, results when the _____ becomes _____.

5. The _____ regulates the amount of light entering the eye while the _____ is important in focusing the light rays onto the _____.

6. The outer-most layer of the eye includes the _____ and the _____. The outer-most layer of the eye is anatomically refers to the _____ _____.

7. Nourishment to the outer retina is provided by the _____.

8. The _____ chamber and _____ chamber collectively is referred to as the _____ segment.

9. A lesion in the _____ nerve results in unilateral blindness while a lesion in the _____ _____ results in bitemporal hemianopia.

10. List the six extra-ocular muscles of the eye.

    _____
    _____
    _____
    _____

11. The muscle _____ _____ is responsible for closing the eyelids while the _____ _____ is responsible for opening the eyelids.

12. List the three (3) most common conditions (diseases) in the United States resulting in blindness. For each of the three condition, identify the anatomical structure effected.

    _____

    _____

    _____

    _____

13. In dark adaptation (in the absence of light), _____, a neurotransmitter, is released _____ (inhibiting/stimulating) the bipolar cells. When light enters the eye, the _____ channels _____, decreasing _____ release resulting in the release of neurotransmitters from the bipolar cells.

14. The _____ fibers of the optic nerve is responsible for the _____ portion of the visual field while the _____ fibers of the optic nerve is responsible for the _____ portion.

15. The primary refractive index of the eye is the _____.

16. The _____ is outer most layer of the eye and is responsible for the attachment of the _____ muscles.

17. The junction between the cornea and the sclera is called the _____.

18. The _____, _____, and _____ belong to the tunica vasculosa of the eye. The _____ _____ connect the ciliary body to the the lens.

19. The _____ _____ is a gelatinous substance found in the _____ segment of the eye. Traction from the this structure can lead to _____ _____ which can lead to vision loss.

20. Define accommodation:

    _____

    _____

    _____

    _____

RESOURCES AND CREDITS

Several anatomy and physiology textbooks have been used as resources for this body of work. The most significant sources are mentioned below. As it is a work in progress suggestions to improve its effectiveness in the cadaver lab are welcome. An initial trial was done with the Nevada State College Honors students by dissecting some regions of the body as outlined in this cadaver guide. The response was positive. It is our hope that it will continue to be a valuable resource among the materials used to learn anatomy efficiently.

1. Drake, Vogl, Mitchell. *Grays Anatomy,* 2nd Edition.
2. Seeley, Steevens and Tate. *Anatomy and Physiology,* 7th & 8th Editions.
3. Martini, N. *Anatomy & Physiology,* 8th Edition.
4. Saladin. *Anatomy & Physiology,* 3rd Edition.
5. Lansen.William's textbook of endocrinology, 10th Edition.
6. Thibodeau & Patton. *Anatomy and Physiology,* 7th Edition.
7. Frederick H. Wezeman. *Essential Companion to Cadaver Dissection,* 2009.
8. University of Wisconsin, Medical School teaching resources.
9. K. Kebede. Cadaver Dissection Guide: The Benjamin Cummings Custom laboratory program for Anatomy & Physiology, Pearson Publishing.
10. Older J. Anatomy: a must for teaching the next generation.Division of Anatomy, Cell and Human Biology, Guy's, School of Biomedical Sciences, Medicine and Dentistry.
11. Andrew Kuniyuki: NSC Cadaver Lab Guidelines.
12. Cadaver Dissection Videos: Lawrence Galtman.
13. McGraw Hill, Anatomy & Physiology Revealed.
14. Martini, Nath. *Fundamentals of Anatomy & Physiology,* 8th Edition.
15. Shier, Butler, Lewis. *Hole's Human Anatomy and Physiology,* 10th Edition.
16. Nielson, G. *Structure and Functions of the Human Body for the Massage Therapist,* 4th Edition.
17. Martini, Timmons, Tallitsch. *Human Anatomy,* 6th Edition.
18. Videos of dissection: The University of Medicine and Dentistry of New Jersey in Stratford.
19. Lecture Notes, Human Cadaver Dissection, Kaskaskia.edu.
20. Cadaver Dissection Videos: University of Michigan, Medical School.
21. Dempster, M., Black, A.McCorry, Wilson, D., Appraisal and Consequences of Cadaver Dissection, Medical Education on line, 2006.
22. O'Carrol R.E., Whiten S., Jackson D., Sinclair D.W. Assessing the emotional impact of cadaver dissection on medical students, Medical Education, 2002.
23. Hancock, D., Williams, M., Taylor, A., Dawson, B, Impact of cadaver dissection on medical students. New Zealand Journal of Psychology, March 01, 2004.
24. Diane J. Cadaver Dissection - Musculocutaneous Nerve, NDS Scientific Research, British Columbia, 2007.
25. Lawrence, G. Video of Cadaver Dissection, Leg and Foot, University of Wisconsin, Medical School.